The morbid anatomy of some of the most important parts of the human body By Matthew Baillie, ...

Matthew Baillie

ECCO

PRINT EDITIONS

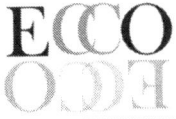

ECCO
Eighteenth Century
Collections Online
Print Editions

Gale ECCO Print Editions

Relive history with *Eighteenth Century Collections Online*, now available in print for the independent historian and collector. This series includes the most significant English-language and foreign-language works printed in Great Britain during the eighteenth century, and is organized in seven different subject areas including literature and language; medicine, science, and technology; and religion and philosophy. The collection also includes thousands of important works from the Americas.

The eighteenth century has been called "The Age of Enlightenment." It was a period of rapid advance in print culture and publishing, in world exploration, and in the rapid growth of science and technology – all of which had a profound impact on the political and cultural landscape. At the end of the century the American Revolution, French Revolution and Industrial Revolution, perhaps three of the most significant events in modern history, set in motion developments that eventually dominated world political, economic, and social life.

In a groundbreaking effort, Gale initiated a revolution of its own: digitization of epic proportions to preserve these invaluable works in the largest online archive of its kind. Contributions from major world libraries constitute over 175,000 original printed works. Scanned images of the actual pages, rather than transcriptions, recreate the works *as they first appeared.*

Now for the first time, these high-quality digital scans of original works are available via print-on-demand, making them readily accessible to libraries, students, independent scholars, and readers of all ages.

For our initial release we have created seven robust collections to form one the world's most comprehensive catalogs of 18th century works.

Initial Gale ECCO Print Editions collections include:

History and Geography
Rich in titles on English life and social history, this collection spans the world as it was known to eighteenth-century historians and explorers. Titles include a wealth of travel accounts and diaries, histories of nations from throughout the world, and maps and charts of a world that was still being discovered. Students of the War of American Independence will find fascinating accounts from the British side of conflict.

Social Science

Delve into what it was like to live during the eighteenth century by reading the first-hand accounts of everyday people, including city dwellers and farmers, businessmen and bankers, artisans and merchants, artists and their patrons, politicians and their constituents. Original texts make the American, French, and Industrial revolutions vividly contemporary.

Medicine, Science and Technology

Medical theory and practice of the 1700s developed rapidly, as is evidenced by the extensive collection, which includes descriptions of diseases, their conditions, and treatments. Books on science and technology, agriculture, military technology, natural philosophy, even cookbooks, are all contained here.

Literature and Language

Western literary study flows out of eighteenth-century works by Alexander Pope, Daniel Defoe, Henry Fielding, Frances Burney, Denis Diderot, Johann Gottfried Herder, Johann Wolfgang von Goethe, and others. Experience the birth of the modern novel, or compare the development of language using dictionaries and grammar discourses.

Religion and Philosophy

The Age of Enlightenment profoundly enriched religious and philosophical understanding and continues to influence present-day thinking. Works collected here include masterpieces by David Hume, Immanuel Kant, and Jean-Jacques Rousseau, as well as religious sermons and moral debates on the issues of the day, such as the slave trade. The Age of Reason saw conflict between Protestantism and Catholicism transformed into one between faith and logic -- a debate that continues in the twenty-first century.

Law and Reference

This collection reveals the history of English common law and Empire law in a vastly changing world of British expansion. Dominating the legal field is the *Commentaries of the Law of England* by Sir William Blackstone, which first appeared in 1765. Reference works such as almanacs and catalogues continue to educate us by revealing the day-to-day workings of society.

Fine Arts

The eighteenth-century fascination with Greek and Roman antiquity followed the systematic excavation of the ruins at Pompeii and Herculaneum in southern Italy; and after 1750 a neoclassical style dominated all artistic fields. The titles here trace developments in mostly English-language works on painting, sculpture, architecture, music, theater, and other disciplines. Instructional works on musical instruments, catalogs of art objects, comic operas, and more are also included.

biblioLife
old books. new life.

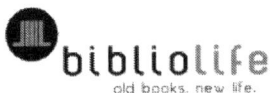

The BiblioLife Network

This project was made possible in part by the BiblioLife Network (BLN), a project aimed at addressing some of the huge challenges facing book preservationists around the world. The BLN includes libraries, library networks, archives, subject matter experts, online communities and library service providers. We believe every book ever published should be available as a high-quality print reproduction; printed on-demand anywhere in the world. This insures the ongoing accessibility of the content and helps generate sustainable revenue for the libraries and organizations that work to preserve these important materials.

The following book is in the "public domain" and represents an authentic reproduction of the text as printed by the original publisher. While we have attempted to accurately maintain the integrity of the original work, there are sometimes problems with the original work or the micro-film from which the books were digitized. This can result in minor errors in reproduction. Possible imperfections include missing and blurred pages, poor pictures, markings and other reproduction issues beyond our control. Because this work is culturally important, we have made it available as part of our commitment to protecting, preserving, and promoting the world's literature.

GUIDE TO FOLD-OUTS MAPS and OVERSIZED IMAGES

The book you are reading was digitized from microfilm captured over the past thirty to forty years. Years after the creation of the original microfilm, the book was converted to digital files and made available in an online database.

In an online database, page images do not need to conform to the size restrictions found in a printed book. When converting these images back into a printed bound book, the page sizes are standardized in ways that maintain the detail of the original. For large images, such as fold-out maps, the original page image is split into two or more pages

Guidelines used to determine how to split the page image follows:

• Some images are split vertically; large images require vertical and horizontal splits.
• For horizontal splits, the content is split left to right.
• For vertical splits, the content is split from top to bottom.
• For both vertical and horizontal splits, the image is processed from top left to bottom right.

THE

MORBID ANATOMY

OF

SOME OF THE MOST IMPORTANT

PARTS

OF THE

HUMAN BODY

BY

MATTHEW BAILLIE, M.D. F.R.S.

FELLOW OF THE ROYAL COLLEGE OF PHYSICIANS, AND
PHYSICIAN OF ST. GEORGE'S HOSPITAL.

LONDON.

PRINTED FOR J. JOHNSON, ST. PAUL'S
CHURCH-YARD; AND G. NICOL,
PALL-MALL.

1793.

TO

SIR GEORGE BAKER, BART.

PRESIDENT,

AND

THE FELLOWS OF THE ROYAL COLLEGE

OF PHYSICIANS,

THIS VOLUME

IS,

WITH THE GREATEST RESPECT,

INSCRIBED

BY THEIR MOST OBEDIENT

HUMBLE SERVANT,

MATTHEW BAILLIE.

PREFACE.

THFRE are some diseases which consist only in morbid actions, but which do not produce any change in the structure of parts: these do not admit of anatomical inquiry after death. There are other diseases, however, where alterations in the structure take place, and these become the proper subjects of anatomical examination.

The object of this work is to explain more minutely than has hitherto been done, the changes of structure arising from morbid actions in some of the most important parts of the human body

This, I hope, will be attended with some advantages to the general science of medicine, and ultimately to its practice. It is

a

very much to be regretted that the knowledge of morbid structure does not certainly
lead to the knowledge of morbid actions,
although the one is the effect of the other;
yet surely it lays the most solid foundation
for prosecuting such inquiries with success.
In proportion, therefore, as we shall become
acquainted with the changes produced in the
structure of parts from diseased actions, we
shall be more likely to make some progress
towards a knowledge of the actions themselves, although it must be very slowly.
The subject in itself is extremely difficult,
because morbid actions are going on in the
minute parts of an animal body excluded
from observation; but still the examination
of morbid structure seems to be one of the
most probable means of throwing light upon it.

Another advantage arising from the more
attentive examination of morbid structure

is, that we shall be able to distinguish between changes which may have some considerable resemblance to each other, and
which have been generally confounded.
This will ultimately lead to a more attentive observation of symptoms while diseased actions are taking place, and be the
means of distinguishing more accurately
diseases. When this has been done, it will
be more likely to produce a successful inquiry after a proper method of treatment.

Another advantage arising from a more
attentive observation of morbid structure is,
that we shall be better fitted to detect diseased alterations in the organization of parts
which are but little, or not at all known.
This will lay the foundation of our inquiry
into the diseases themselves, so that we shall
add to our knowledge of the pathology of
the body, and perhaps also to our knowledge of remedies.

A third advantage still from observing attentively morbid structure is, that theories taken up hastily about diseases will be occasionally corrected   The human mind is prone to form opinions upon every subject which is presented to it, but from a natural indolence is frequently averse to inquire into the circumstances which can alone form a sufficient ground for them   This is the most general cause of false opinions, which have not only pervaded medicine, but every other branch of knowledge When, however, the mind shall be obliged to observe facts which cannot be reconciled with such opinions, it will be the best means of shewing that they are unfounded, and of making them be laid aside   We grant, it does not always happen that men are induced to give up their opinions, or even to think them wrong, upon observing facts which do not agree with them, but surely it is the best means of producing this effect ; and whatever change may be wrought on the individuals themselves, the world will be convinced, who have fewer prejudices to combat.

A person who previously had attended very accurately to symptoms, but was unacquainted with the disease, when he comes to examine the body after death, and finds some of the appearances that are described in this Treatise, will acquire a knowledge of the whole disease. He will be able to guide himself on such knowledge in similar cases, and also to inform others. It may, perhaps, too, lead him to a proper method of treatment.

When a person has become well acquainted with diseased appearances, he will be better able to make his remarks, in examining dead bodies, so as to judge more accurately how far the symptoms and appearances agree with each other ; he will be able also to give a more distinct account of what he has observed, so that his data shall become a more accurate ground of reasoning for others.

The natural structure of the different parts of the human body has been very minutely examined, so that anatomy may be said to have arrived at a high pitch of perfection ; but our knowledge of the changes of structure produced by disease, which may be called the Morbid Anatomy, is still very imperfect. Such changes have commonly been observed only in their more obvious appearances, and very seldom with much minuteness or accuracy of discrimination.

Any works explaining morbid structure which I have seen, are very different in their plan from the present : they either consist of cases containing an account of

diseases and dissections collected together
in periodical publications, without any natural connection among each other; or
consist of very large collections of cases, ar-
ranged according to some order. In some
of these periodical works, the diseased
structure has been frequently explained
with a sufficient degree of accuracy, but in
all the larger works it has been often described too generally. The descriptions too
of the principal diseased appearances have
been sometimes obscured, by taking notice
of smaller collateral circumstances, which
had no connection with them or the diseases from whence they arose. Both of
these faults even too frequently occur in
the stupendous work of Morgagni de Causis
et Sedibus Morborum, upon which, when
considered in all its parts, it would be difficult to bestow too high praise · besides,
the bulk of these very large collections pre-

vents them from being generally in the possession of practitioners, and also renders then more difficult to consult.

In the present work we propose to give no cases; but simply an account of the morbid changes of structure which take place in the thoracic and abdominal viscera, in the organs of generation in both sexes, and in the brain This will be done according to a local arrangement, very much in the same manner as if we were describing natural structure, and will be accompanied with observations upon morbid actions which may occasionally arise My situation has given me more than the ordinary opportunities of examining morbid structure. Dr. Hunter's collection contains a very large number of preparations exhibiting morbid appearances, which I can have recourse to at any time for examination. Being physician to a large hospital, and engaged in teaching

anatomy, I have also very frequent opportunities of examining diseases in dead
bodies. What this work will contain will
be principally an account of what I have
seen myself; but I shall also take advantage
of what has been observed by others. This
work is intended to comprehend an account
of the most common, as well as many of
the very rare appearances of disease in the
vital and more important parts of the human body. It is evident from the nature
of this work, that it must be progressive:
some appearances of disease will be observed in future, with which we are at present
totally unacquainted, and others which we
know very little of now, will afterwards
be known perfectly.

The principal motive which has induced
me to undertake this work, is to render the
morbid structure of parts more accurately
and generally known, as one of the best

means of advancing our knowledge of diseases.

Although I have ventured to lay this work before the Public, yet I am very sensible of its imperfections. There are some appearances described which I have only had an opportunity of seeing once, and which, therefore, may be supposed to be described less fully and exactly than if I had been able to make repeated examinations. There are others which I have seen long before I had any idea of undertaking this work, and which I may be supposed to have observed less accurately than if there had been a particular object in view There are others still, which I have only had an opportunity of examining in preparations. In some of these, certain appearances may be supposed to be lost, which might have been observed had they been examined recently after death. All of these are sources of inaccuracy, which may be said in some degree to be unavoidable. I have endeavoured, however, to be accurate; and if the Public should approve of the plan of this work, I shall be very careful, by the addition of new materials, and by repeated observations, to render it more perfect.

CONTENTS.

CHAPTER I.

CHAPTER II.

CHAPTER III.

CHAPTER IV.

CHAPTER V.

CHAPTER VI.

Diseased Appearances within the Cavity of the Abdomen.

Ascites — Inflammation of the Perito-

CHAPTER XV.

CHAPTER XVI.

CHAPTER XVII.

CHAPTER XVIII.

CHAPTER XIX.

CHAPTER XX.

CHAPTER XXI.

CHAPTER XXII

CHAPTER XXIII.

The Hymen imperforated—The Clitoris enlarged— The Nymphæ enlarged— The external Labia growing together.

CHAPTER XXIV.

Inflammation of the Dura Mater—Adhesions — Pus formed—Gangrene— Scrofulous Tumours connected with the Dura Mater—Spongy Tumours growing from the Dura Mater— Bony Matter formed in the Dura Mater—Very strong Adhesion of the Dura Mater to the Cranium—Diseased Appearances of the Tunica Arachnoides—Veins of the Pia Mater turgid with Blood—The Pia Mater inflamed

CHAPTER I.

Diseased Appearances of the Pericardium.

THE pericardium, or the membrane which surrounds the heart like a bag, and is reflected upon its surface, giving it a smooth external covering, is liable to inflammation. This is not a very common disease, although it happens sufficiently often to afford frequent opportunities of examining its effects after death. The disease, from its nature, cannot be confined to any particular periods of life, yet from what I have seen, I should believe that it takes place more commonly when the body has for some time arrived at the adult state, than either in childhood or in advanced age

In inflammation of the pericardium, the membrane is frequently thicker than in its natural state, and I think is also a little more pulpy. This change depends upon additional matter being thrown into the membrane by the increased action of the small vessels which are distributed upon it. It is also crowded with a very unusual number of minute vessels, which contain a florid blood, and which form various junctions with each other. Upon the inside of the pericardium, there is a layer of a yellowish pulpy matter, which commonly does not adhere firmly to it, but may be easily separated. It generally extends over the whole of its inner surface, and varies a good deal in its thickness. In some instances it is as thin as a wafer, and in others as thick as a half crown. In this matter which is lining the pericardium, there is frequently to be seen a slight red appearance from small blood vessels which are ramifying through it, but these are most distinctly detected by fine injection

These vessels, however, are sometimes numerous, and may be traced passing from the
pericardium into the pulpy matter; and I
have also seen in it small spots of a florid
blood. This circumstance becomes a very
convincing proof of this extravasated matter possessing a living principle; for one
cannot imagine that blood vessels would
shoot into, and ramify through, a substance
which is dead. * Upon its inner surface, this
matter very frequently throws out little irregular laminated projections, giving the appearance of a lace work, and junctions are
often formed between that portion of it lining
the pericardium, which is reflected like a
bag, and that other portion lying upon the
pericardium, which is the immediate covering of the heart. This matter has a very close
resemblance, both in colour and structure, to
the coagulable lymph of the blood, and is
probably nothing else than this substance
separated from the blood by a peculiar action
of the small vessels of the pericardium

* This is an argument used by Mr Hunter, in support
of the living principle of the blood.

At the same time that this layer of pulpy matter is thrown out upon the inner surface of the pericardium, there is accumulated in its cavity, more or less of a brownish or yellowish fluid. There is sometimes only a few ounces of it ; at other times more than a pint. In it there are floating loose shreds of the pulpy matter formerly explained, and there is also occasionally some mixture of pus This fluid resembles in its properties the serum of the blood, and has commonly been considered as the serum. It is probably separated in part from the coagulable lymph while it forms the solid layer, on the inside of the pericardium, similar to the spontaneous separation of the different parts of the blood after bleeding ; but I should believe that it was not wholly accumulated in this manner, because it is often in very large proportion to the quantity of the coagulable lymph. Inflammation of the pericardium sometimes advances to form pus, although rarely. Of this I have seen one instance. The pericardium was very much thickened, was inflamed, and lined with coagulable lymph, but there was no sign of ulceration in any part of it. This last circumstance will be more particularly noticed, when we come to speak of the diseased appearances of the pleura. The pericardium in this case, contained more than a quart of common pus. When the pericardium is inflamed which forms the immediate covering of the heart, the muscular substance of the latter is occasionally inflamed to some depth.

Adhesions of the Pericardium to the Heart.

In opening dead bodies, adhesions of the pericardium to the heart, are not uncommonly found. The adhesion is sometimes at different spots; at other times is extended over the whole surface. It either consists of a thin membrane, or of a more solid matter. When it is a thin membrane, it resembles very much, the common cellular membrane of the body, and when the matter is solid, it differs little from the coagulable lymph of the blood. Whether the adhesion be in the one way or the other, the matter of the adhesion is in both cases capable of being rendered vascular from injection. The adhesion too, is in both cases formed from the pulpy matter formerly explained, for I have oftener than once had an opportunity of tracing its gradual changes into each. Such adhesions are to be considered as the consequence of previous inflammation, and shew that an inflammation of the pericardium may be survived. They connect the pericardium in different cases, more closely or loosely to the surface of the heart, and where the connection is close, the inflammation has probably been more recent; where it is loose the inflammation has probably been of older date, so that time has been given for the adhesions to be elongated by the motion of the heart. It is worthy of remark that where there is an adhesion of the pericardium to the heart, the latter sometimes pulsates so violently, that it is impossible to distinguish it from the pulsation of an aneurism.

Dropsy of the Pericardium.

This disease is not uncommon, and I believe is most frequent at an advanced period of life. I have seen it however in persons considerably under the age of thirty; and it probably also happens occasionally in childhood. I have seen oftener than once both anasarca and ascites in children under twelve years old, which is as improbable as the accumulation of water in the pericardium. Water is sometimes found accumulated in the pericardium, while there is none in any other cavity; but generally it is accompanied with the accumulation of water in the other cavities of the thorax.

This water varies a good deal in quantity, amounting in some cases hardly to two ounces, and in others to more than a pint. Although the quantity be large which may

happen to be accumulated, yet I do not recollect to have seen the pericardium very
much stretched, but it has always appeared
as if it could contain a greater quantity. It
is probable therefore that the pericardium
may really grow so as to keep pace with
the accumulation.

The fluid which is accumulated, is of a
brown colour, having a darker or lighter
shade in different cases, and resembles in its
properties the serum of the blood. If the
person should happen at the same time to
have jaundice, then the fluid has a pretty
deep yellow tinge from bile. It has however frequently a yellowish colour, like the
serum, without there being any reason to
suppose that bile has been circulating with
the blood.

The accumulation of water in the cavity
of the pericardium, may proceed from two
causes.

The one is, that the small exhalant
vessels opening upon the inner surface of the
pericardium, may throw out an unusually

large quantity of fluid into its cavity, which is not absorbed in the same proportion by the absorbent vessels of that part : the other is, that the fluid may be thrown into the cavity in the natural quantity, but may not be absorbed in the natural proportion, from a defect in the action of the absorbent vessels.

I once had an opportunity of seeing two or three scrofulous tumours, growing within the cavity of the pericardium, one of which was nearly as large as a walnut. They consisted of a white soft matter, somewhat resembling curd, or new cheese. The pericardium is a very unusual part of the body to be attacked by scrofula, and therefore this must be a very rare appearance of disease The tumours had probably been slow in their progress, as in scrofula generally, and this disease could not have been guessed at in the living body.

I have twice found (and it has been seen much oftener by an anatomist * of the best authority) the pericardium so changed as to

* Mr. Hunter

resemble a common ox's bladder in some degree dried, or like a common pericardium which had been for some time exposed to the air As the thorax and abdomen, were entire in both cases, no opening whatever having been made into either, this effect could not arise from evaporation. Were this capable of taking place, the appearance here noticed, would be very usual in examining dead bodies, and the internal parts generally would be affected by the influence of the same cause It must be considered therefore as the effect of a process which was going on during life. The cause of this appearance is probably a defect in the action of the exhalant vessels of the pericardium, so that the fluid which naturally lubricates this part, was not secreted in the proper quantity There is nothing more difficult to conceive in this, than a defect in the action of any other part of the body.

A portion of the pericardium has in some instances, been observed to be converted

into cartilage,* and in others into bone,†
but both of these changes are very uncommon.

* See Morgagni de Causis et Sedibus morborum, Epist.
XXII. Art. 10.

† See Bonetus, Tom. 1, p. 583.

CHAP. II.

Diseased Appearances of the Heart.

INFLAMMATION of the substance of the heart is a rare disease, and is most commonly connected with an inflammation of the pericardium. When the pericardium covering its surface is inflamed, the inflammation sometimes passes a little way into the substance of the heart. That part of it becomes much more crowded with small vessels than in its natural state, and there are sometimes to be seen a few spots of extravasated blood. The substance of the heart may however be inflamed without inflammation of the pericardium   I recollect an instance of this sort where no marks of inflammation could be observed in that membrane, but where there was a little more water than usual accumulated in its cavity.   In this case the pulsation had been so strong, that it was impossible to distinguish it from the pulsation of an aneurism. Authors have mentioned cases of abscesses and ulcers * of the heart, but these I am persuaded are extremely rare. It happens still more rarely that the heart becomes mortified, although this diseased state of it has also been observed.†

In opening dead bodies there is very often to be seen upon the surface of the heart, a white opaque spot, like a thickening of the pericardium. This is sometimes not broader than a sixpence; at other times as broad as a crown. It is most commonly on the surface of the right ventricle, and is very rarely to be seen either on the surface of the left ventricle, or of the auricles, although it is occasionally on both.

It consists of an adventitious membrane, formed on a portion of the pericardium

* Vid. Morgagni, Epist XXV. Artic 17   Vid. Bonet, Tom 1, p 849; and also Lieutaud, Tom 2, p. 27.

† Vid. Lieutaud, Tom 2, p 33.

which covers the heart, and may easily be dissected off so as to leave the pericardium entire. It is an appearance, I believe, of no consequence whatever, and is so very common that it can hardly be considered as a disease.

Polypus.

This has been considered by the older anatomists, as a very common and a very fatal disease. By many of the moderns it has been rejected as a disease altogether. It consists in a mass of the coagulable lymph filling up some of the large cavities of the heart, particularly the ventricles, and extending into the neighbouring large vessels. The coagulable lymph is of a yellowish white colour, sometimes of a very yellow colour, and has considerable firmness. It fills up the cavity completely, or nearly so, in which it is found; and in the ventricles it shoots out processes between the fasciculi of the muscular fibres From this circumstance, probably, it has derived its name. It also extends into the large arteries which arise from the ventricles, and is often moulded to the shape of the semi-lunar valves at their origin. Any examples of this appearance which it has occurred to me to observe, have been chiefly in preparations, and had undoubtedly taken place after death. In order that the circulation may be carried on it is necessary that the cavities of the heart be free for the transmission of blood; and if any one of its cavities should be plugged up, the circulation would necessarily be stopped altogether A polypus, however, plugs up the cavity of the heart in which it is formed so entirely as to prevent the circulation. It may be said perhaps, that polypi are formed gradually, and the circulation is carried on for some time, although very imperfectly. We have no general evidence however of coagula of blood being formed in the ordinary circulation where there is a healthy structure of the parts concerned in this function.

When polypi are examined, there is the same sort of appearance through their whole substance, which shews that the whole coagulum had been formed at the same time. Both of those circumstances seem to contradict very strongly the opinion that polypi are formed during life. When polypi are formed, I believe that the coagulation of the blood does not take place very quickly after death. They are without any admixture of the red globules of blood, and therefore the blood has been sufficiently long in coagulating to allow these globules to separate from the other parts in consequence of their greater specific gravity.

The ordinary coagulations of the blood, which commonly do not fill up very fully the cavities of the heart (although instances occasionally occur of this sort) take place pretty soon after death, because the red particles of the blood are generally arrested in the coagulum. It may be worth while to remark, that there is sometimes found a portion of a coagulum in one of the ventricles of a yellow colour, and with an oily appearance so as to resemble exactly fat. There is however no admixture of oil in it, and it possesses all the ordinary properties of the coagulable lymph. The colour of a coagulum sometimes depends on a portion of bile having circulated with the blood during life, as in cases of jaundice; but it takes place also when there is no reason to suppose that bile is mixed with the blood. These appearances depend probably on certain circumstances of the coagulation; but what those circumstances are, it is very difficult to determine.

It sometimes happens, although I believe very rarely, that the heart becomes aneurismal This disease consists in a part of it being dilated into a pouch, which is commonly more or less filled with coagulated blood. Of this disease I have only seen one instance. The apex of the left ventricle was dilated into a pouch large enough to contain a small orange, was much thinner than in the healthy structure, and was lined

C

with a thick white opaque membrane.
There was hardly contained in it any coagulated blood; but the quantity of the coagulated blood depends commonly on the
size of the bag.

This disease most probably arose from
the muscular structure at the apex of the
ventricle becoming weaker than in any
other part, so that when the ventricle contracted upon the blood it was pushed against
the weakened part, which was not fully able
to resist its impetus, and therefore was gradually dilated. Had the strength of the a-
pex of the left ventricle been in due proportion to that of the other parts, it is impossible that the aneurismal swelling should
ever have taken place.

The most frequent situation of aneurism
within the cavity of the thorax, is at the
arch of the aorta. In this disease the arch
of the aorta, is much enlarged beyond its
usual size, sometimes forming an uniform
tumour, and at other times there are smaller
aneurismal swellings rising out of the

larger one. This enlargement of the artery, if very considerable, is more or less filled
with coagulated blood, which is disposed in
concentric laminæ. The coats of the dilated artery, are nearly of the same thickness
with those in its natural state, and therefore
in proportion as the swelling increases, new
matter must be deposited in the coats of the
artery. This new matter is undoubtedly
deposited with a view to prevent the artery
from being so soon ruptured as it would be ·
otherwise, and is formed by the action of
the vasa vasorum. A portion of the new
matter may perhaps also be formed by the
action of the parts immediately in contact
with the artery.

The coats of the artery, both at the place
where the aneurism is formed, and near it,
are considerably altered from their natural
structure. They are more readily divisible
into different layers, and have often formed
in them spots of bony matter. These spots
are frequently of a yellowish colour, and
are formed either in the internal mem-

brane of the artery or immediately behind
it.

The coats of the artery in the neighbourhood of the aneurism, are often found to be
very irregular in their texture, being in
some places transparent and thin, in others
thick and opaque ; and there is sometimes
the appearance of a double internal membrane.   The same sort of structure is also
to be found in the coats of the aneurism itself.   The arteries near an aneurism are
diseased to a greater or less extent in different persons, but I do not recollect one instance in which they were totally free from
disease

The disease sometimes ends fatally, by
the enlarged artery bursting, and the blood
escaping into the cavity of the pericardium;
but it very often has a further progress;
the swelling of the aneurism gradually increases till at length it presses against the
sternum, and the cartilaginous extremities
of some of the ribs   This pressure occasions a portion of the sternum and the ribs

to be absorbed, and the tumour is thereby perceived externally. This absorption of the sternum and ribs is not accompanied with the formation of pus, but is a process which is insensibly taking place according to the extent of the pressure. The tumour gradually increases in size, till perhaps it is as large as a child's head at birth ; the skin then becomes in some measure dead, and cracks from distention at the highest point of the tumour, a portion of the coagulated blood is forced out by the impetus of the circulation, and the person is cut off instantaneously. The blood sometimes oozes out slowly, and the person sinks gradually under its loss.

Aneurisms at the arch of the aorta, as well as in every other part of the arterial system, arise from the coats of the artery being previously diseased, which are thereby unable to resist sufficiently the impetus of blood that strikes against them. This is obvious both from the diseased structure of the coats of an aneurism it-

self, and of the artery in its neighbourhood.

I have also found very frequently diseased appearances in the arch of the aorta,
which were not advanced far enough to
produce aneurism. These consist in little
white opaque spots, being formed in the
inner membrane of the artery, and its coats
are more easily separable from each other
than in the healthy state.

The reason why aneurisms take place
more frequently in the arch of the aorta,
than in any other part of the arterial system, is its curvature, which exposes it to the
full impetus of the blood propelled by the
strength of the left ventricle. Aneurisms
hardly ever happen in the pulmonary artery, because there is no arch formed by the
pulmonary artery, and the blood readily
passes by two large branches into the substance of the lungs. It may not be improbable too, that the pulmonary artery may
not be so liable as the aorta to those diseased
alterations of structure, upon which aneurism ultimately depends.

Aneurisms in the arch of the aorta, as well as in every other part of the arterial system, happen much more rarely in women than in men. This arises from two causes. The one is, that women, from their sedentary life, are less liable to an increased impetus of the blood, occasioned by excited circulation ; the other is, that the arteries in this sex appear to be less liable to diseased alterations of structure. This is not at all peculiar to aneurism, some other diseases prevail in the one sex from which the other is in a great measure exempt.

The time of life at which aneurisms are most frequent, seems to be about the middle age. When very strong pulsation is to be felt of the heart, we are not always to consider the disease as aneurism, especially if the person be young and of the female sex. I have known an instance where an adhesion of the pericardium to the heart, was attended with that very strong pulsation which is usual in aneurism ; and I have known another instance where there was an unusually strong pulsation at the time the heart was a little inflamed upon its surface, and there was a small quantity of water in the pericardium.

The three semi-lunar valves at the origin of the aorta, or of the pulmonary artery, are often found diseased. This consists in the deposition of a bony or earthy matter. When a small portion of this bony or earthy matter is deposited, the valves are only somewhat impaired in their function, but when the quantity of matter is considerable, they must lose their valvular function altogether. The communication between the ventricles and the arteries, becomes very narrow, the circulation is extremely interrupted, and the person is at length destroyed. This disease most commonly takes place towards an advanced period of life, but I have seen an instance of it in a boy of ten years old.

It sometimes happens that the semi-lunar valves are considerably thickened, and of an opaque white colour: in this case the

coats of the artery in the neighbourhood I
believe are commonly thickened and diseased

There is a preparation in Dr. Hunter's
collection, where one of the semi-lunar valves is thickened, having at the same time
little tenacity, and being of a brown colour,
in which a considerable rupture had taken
place. It is very rare that such an occurrence happens, and in the present instance
the rupture was so large that I believe it
must have proved very soon fatal.

The valvular apparatus between the auricles and ventricles, is liable to the formation of bony and earthy matter, as well as
the valves which are situated at the origin
of the two large arteries, but by no means
so frequently. What this depends upon it
is very difficult to determine. These valves may perhaps be considered as belonging more to the veinal than the arterial system, and it is very certain that ossification
takes place very seldom in veins, although
very often in arteries.

The valvular apparatus between the auricles and ventricles, is also occasionally thickened, having lost all its transparency, and having an opaque white colour. The chordæ tendineæ are also thicker than natural ; and the internal membrane lining the ventricles, is frequently at the same time a good deal thickened, appearing like a firm white membrane. Under such circumstances the heart is often found to be considerably enlarged beyond its usual size. I have also seen the valvular apparatus between the auricle and the ventricle, in a state of inflammation, and covered with a layer of coagulable lymph. This I believe to be very uncommon

It sometimes happens, and I believe chiefly in those who are advanced in life, that the heart at some part becomes thinner, and upon any great exertion bursts. The blood escapes into the cavity of the pericardium, and the person is instantly destroyed.

Of such cases I have seen one instance only, but have heard from the best authotity of another. They both happened to men ; and I mention this circumstance because men appear to be more subject to diseases of the heart and blood vessels than women. It is probable that persons dying from this cause, have on account of the suddenness of their death been supposed to die of apoplexy.

Cases have occurred, although very rarely, in which a large quantity of blood has been accumulated in the cavity of the pericardium, but where no rupture could be discovered after the most diligent search, either in the heart itself, or in any of its vessels. This appears very wonderful, and not at all what any person would expect a priori. Upon the supposition of there being no rupture, two conjectures only have occurred to me with regard to the possibility of such an effect taking place, and they are both attended with considerable difficulty.

The one is, that the vessels upon the surface of the heart, may have lost a part of the compactness of their texture, so that the blood may have escaped through their coats by transudation. The other is, that blood may have been thrown out by the extremi-ties of the small vessels opening upon the surface, of that portion chiefly of the pericardium which forms the immediate covering of the heart, whose orifices may have been to a very uncommon degree relaxed.*

It also happens, although I believe very rarely, that a heart is so imperfectly formed as to allow of life being continued for some length of time in a very uncomfortable state, but to be ultimately the cause of death. There are two cases of this sort described by the late Dr. Hunter,† and there is one specimen of this malformation preserved in his collection The malformation preserved in the collection, consists in the right ventricle of the heart being extremely small, and the pulmonary artery being very small also which arises from it. At its origin

* See Med. Observations, Vol. 4, p 330 Memoirs of Med. Society, Vol 1, p. 238
† Vid. Medical Observations, Vol 6, p 291.

from the right ventricle it is completely
impervious. The ductus arteriosus is open,
but forms likewise a small canal, and terminates in the left branch of the pulmonary
artery. The right auricle is larger than its
natural size, probably from the frequent
accumulation of blood in it; and the communication between the two auricles, by
means of the foramen ovale, is much larger
than usual. The child in whom this mal-
formation was found, had its skin of a very
dark colour, had very laborious respiration,
and violent action of the heart. It lived
only thirteen days.

In another case related by Dr. Hunter,
the pulmonary artery was very small, especially at its origin, and there was a deficiency
in the septum cordis, at the basis of the
heart, large enough to allow a small thumb
to pass through it. The person in whom
this malformation of the heart was found,
lived about thirteen years. He never had
a fresh complexion, but it was always dark,

or tending to black. He was often seized with fits, especially when there was any hurry upon his spirits, or there had been any brisk motion of his body.

It is obvious that in these deviations from the natural structure, too small a quantity of blood must pass through the lungs to receive the benefit of respiration, and this will be more or less according to the degree of the deviation. The blood will from this cause be of a dark colour, as it is well known that it receives the florid hue from the influence of the air upon it in the lungs. Hence the colour of the skin must be necessarily sallow or dark, and this will be increased when the blood is more than usual accumulated in the veins. It is natural to think that in such structures of the heart, the circulation will be carried on with much more difficulty when it is excited beyond its usual standard. This may even be increased to such a degree that the circulation must for a short time be suspended altogether. It was from this cause probably that fits occasionally were produced, as related in one of the cases.

There is an example also in Dr. Hunter's collection of a heart from a child, which had a hole in the septum ventriculorum at the basis of the heart, large enough to allow a goose quill readily to pass through it. The child was still-born at six months, and the hole in the septum evidently arose from o-riginal malformation. This too, is descri-bed by Dr. Hunter, in the sixth volume of the Medical Observations. An instance somewhat similar to this has likewise been published by Dr. Pulteney, in the third vo-lume of the Medical Transactions, where the person to whom this monstrosity belonged, lived to near fourteen years of age.

I do not know how far I ought to men-tion, consistently with the plan of this pub-lication, that the heart is sometimes found of a very uncommon size, but without any disease in its structure. This occasionally takes place, and perhaps should properly be considered as a monstrous formation.

In most instances however where the heart is a good deal enlarged beyond its usual size, without any external morbid appearance belonging to it, I am persuaded that the valves between the auricles and ventricles will be found thickened from disease.

Hydatids * have occasionally been found adhering to the heart, but I have myself met with no instances of this sort. They do not appear to be of the same kind in every part of the body, but their nature I will explain particularly when I come to describe the diseased appearances of the liver and kidneys.

A portion of the heart has been observed to be converted into bone.† Earthy matter has also been found deposited in the muscular substance of the heart.‡ None of those appearances have come under my own observation, and they are to be looked upon as very uncommon

* See Morgagni, Epist. XXV. Art. 15.

† See Morgagni, Epist XXVII Art. 16 ; see also Medical Communications, Vol. 1, p. 228.

‡ See Bonetus, Tom. 1, p. 820, and p. 825.

CHAP. III.

Diseased Appearances in the Cavity of the Thorax.

Inflammation.

THE pleura, or the membrane which lines the cavity of the thorax, is very subject to inflammation. This may take place at any period of life, but it is more frequent at the age when the body is just arrived at the adult state, and all its actions are carried on with vigour, than either in childhood or in advanced age. The pleura appears to be more liable to inflammation than any membrane lining those cavities which have no external opening, as the peritonæum, the tunica vaginalis testis, and some others. Why this should be the case, it is perhaps difficult to determine. The branches of the intercostal vessels, which are very numerous, piercing through the substance of the inter-

D

costal muscles, communicate a good deal by
anastomosis with the external vessels on the
sides of the chest Hence whatever may act
upon these external vessels, so as to excite
contraction in them, may be supposed capable of producing an accumulation of
blood, as well as an increased action in the
inner branches of the intercostals, many of
which are distributed upon the pleura. Perhaps, too, upon another principle, there
may be a greater consent between the action
of the external and internal vessels of the
chest, than in the body generally. If these
observations be just, they would account for
the very frequent inflammation of the pleura ; but they are only to be considered in
the light of a conjecture Whatever be the
cause of it, the fact is undoubted that the
pleura is more liable to inflammation than
any other membrane investing cavities
which have no external opening. This is
so much the case that one can hardly examine the chest of any person who has arrived at the adult state, without perceiving

more or less the traces of present or former inflammation.

When the pleura is inflamed, it becomes thicker than it is naturally, and in some degree pulpy. There is also interspersed through it a great number of very small vessels containing florid blood, and a layer of coagulable lymph, is at the same time thrown out upon its surface. This layer is sometimes very thin, and at other times of considerable thickness. It is either smooth upon its surface, or it throws out many fine small flocculi, which exhibit the appearance of a rich lace work There is also poured into the cavity of the thorax a serous fluid, in which are floating many small broken laminæ of the coagulable lymph; and there is occasionally some mixture of pus.

The coagulable lymph, covering the pleura which forms the external membrane of the lungs, frequently adheres to that which covers the pleura that is reflected on the inside of the ribs and the intercostal spaces, either in small portions, or by extended surfaces. Upon such occasions I have sometimes been able to trace the gradual change of the adhesion from the nature of coagulable lymph to that of cellular membrane. This coagulable lymph is capable of being rendered vascular from injection, as we have already mentioned in the inflammation of the pericardium. When the pleura is inflamed which covers the lungs, the substance of the latter is frequently inflamed to some depth.

Adhesions in the Cavity of the Thorax.

Adhesions are often found between that portion of the pleura which covers the lungs, and that other portion of it which lines the ribs and the intercostal spaces, while there is no sign whatever of present inflammation. These adhesions are often partial, and then they are most commonly to be found at the upper and posterior part of the chest ; but they are sometimes extended over the whole

cavity. They either connect the parts together closely, and then they often consist
of a firm thick membrane, or they connect
them loosely, when they consist of a soft
spungy membrane, which exactly resembles
the common cellular membrane of the body.
Such adhesions are the consequence of inflammation, and are perhaps the most common morbid appearance to be found in dead
bodies

Empyema.

Pus is not unfrequently found accumulated in the cavity of the chest, forming the
disease called empyema. This may either
arise from the blood vessels of the pleura
being in such a state of inflammation as to
form pus, or from the bursting of some abscess in the lungs, so as to evacuate its pus
into the cavity of the thorax. When pus
is formed by an inflamed state of the pleura,
there is no occasion for ulceration to take
place The pleura is found entire, but is
covered with a layer of the coagulable

lymph. This fact has been long ago ascertained by the late Dr. Hunter. The formation of the pus depends on a certain state of action in the vessels of the pleura. The pus may either be accumulated in the whole cavity of the chest, or may be confined to a part of it by adhesions taking place between the lungs and the pleura, which invests the ribs and the intercostal spaces. When pus is evacuated into the cavity of the chest by the bursting of an abscess in the lungs, it is almost always confined within certain limits by adhesions. In cases of empyema, there is frequently no particular appearance of the chest observable on the outside: there is sometimes however a fullness to be perceived externally on the side where the matter is accumulated, and even occasionally an evident swelling between two of the ribs, as of matter pointing Ulceration has also been known to take place in one or more of the intercostal spaces, so that the matter has been evacuated externally. There is an example in Dr Hunter's collection, where the matter had been evacuated from the chest by a great many openings in the intercostal spaces.

Hydrothorax.

A watery fluid is not uncommonly found in one or both cavities of the chest, forming the disease called hydrothorax. It is often attended with the accumulation of water in other parts of the body, especially in the pericardium, and the cellular membrane of the lower extremities. The fluid in hydrothorax is commonly of a brown or yellowish colour, but occasionally has a red colour arising from the mixture of the red globules of blood. It resembles in its properties the serum. It is found to vary a good deal in quantity in different cases, sometimes amounting only to a few ounces, and at other times to several quarts. When it is accumulated in very large quantity in either side of the chest, that side appears to be fuller to the eye externally, and when the cavity is laid open after death, the lungs on that side are found more or less com-

pressed. I have seen a lung so compressed, as not to be larger than the closed fist.

Water is likewise found in the cavity of
the chest where there are considerable adhesions. This shews that a good deal of
inflammation had formerly taken place,
which had probably, by throwing out a
considerable quantity of serum, laid the
foundation of the hydrothorax.*

Ossification of the Pleura.

It sometimes happens, although I believe
rarely, that a portion of the pleura is converted into bone. This consists of a thin
plate, and sometimes extends over a pretty
broad surface of the pleura. In all the cases
which I have seen, the bony matter seemed
to me to be exactly like ordinary bone. I
have never seen it form a thick irregular knob,
but always a thin plate. The cause which
first excites this diseased process it is very

* This circumstance is illustrated in several instances
by Mr Cruikshank, in his Treatise upon the Absorbent
System. See 2d edition, p 116.

difficult to determine; but there can be no
doubt that the bone is formed by the small
vessels of the pleura, taking on the same
mode of action which vessels do in the formation of ordinary bone. This process is not
peculiar to the pleura, but takes place in almost every part of the body: I believe, however, that it is more common in the pleura
than in any other similar membrane. In the
cases which I have observed, this process
seemed not to have been attended with
much inconvenience. There was no inflammation found in the pleura surrounding the
bone, nor in the substance of the lungs under it   One could imagine, however, if the
bone were to grow irregularly, so as to form
pretty sharp processes, that it might excite
inflammation, and lay the foundation of a
fatal disease.

CHAP. IV.

Diseased Appearances of the Lungs.

Inflammation.

INFLAMMATION of the substance of the
lungs, I believe, seldom takes place without
some similar affection of the pleura; at
least in the instances which I have seen, this
has been most frequently the case. When
a portion of the lungs is inflamed, its spungy
structure appears much redder than usual,
the colour being partly florid and partly
of a darker hue. This arises from a much
greater number of small vessels than usual,
being distributed upon the cells of the lungs
which are capable of admitting the red globules of the blood. There is also an extravasation of the coagulable lymph into the
substance of the lungs, and sometimes of
blood. The extravasated blood has been
said upon some occasions to be in very large

quantity; but this has never fallen under my own observation.

In consequence of the greater quantity of blood being accumulated in the inflamed portion of the lungs, they become considerably heavier, and will frequently sink in water. The pleura covering the inflamed portion of the lungs has generally a similar affection; it is crowded with fine red vessels, and has generally lying upon it a layer of coagulable lymph.

This inflamed state of the lungs is to be distinguished from blood accumulated in some part of them after death in consequence of gravitation   From the body lying in the horizontal posture after death, blood is often accumulated at the posterior part of the lungs, giving them there a deeper colour, and rendering them heavier.   In this case there will be found no crowd of fine vessels filled with blood, nor any other mark of inflammation of the pleura. Where blood too is accumulated in any part of a lung after death from gravitation, it is always of a dark colour ; but where blood is accumulated from inflammation, portions of the inflamed part will appear florid.

It is very common to find abscesses form-ed in the lungs. These sometimes consist of small cavities containing pus, and at other times the cavities are very large, so that the greater part of the substance of the lungs has been destroyed These cavities some-times communicate only with branches of the trachea, which are destroyed in the pro-gress of the ulceration; at other times they open into the cavity of the chest, emptying their contents there, and forming the disease which is called empyema Where abscesses are deeply seated in the substance of the lungs, the pleura is commonly not affected; but where abscesses are formed near the sur-face, it is almost constantly inflamed. The lungs round the boundaries of an abscess, when it has arisen from common inflamma-tion, are more solid in their texture, in con-sequence of coagulable lymph being thrown out during the progress of the inflammation.

When the abscesses are scrofulous, the texture of the lungs in the neighbourhood is sometimes not firmer than usual, but presents the common natural appearance This I believe to be principally the case when the abscesses are small, and placed at a considerable distance from each other. When a portion of the lungs is crowded with tubercles, and some of these are converted into abscesses, the intermediate substance of the lungs is often of a very solid texture. When blood vessels are traced into an abscess of the lungs, I have found them, upon examination, very much contracted, just before they reach the abscess, so that the opening of their extremities has been closed up entirely On such occasions it will require a probe to be pushed with a good deal of force, in order to open again their extremities The late ingenious Dr. Stark,* has found in some of these vessels, the blood coagulated This change in the blood vessels is no doubt with a view to prevent large

* See Dr Stark's works, p. 28

hæmorrhages from taking place, which
would certainly be almost immediately fatal.

When abscesses of the lungs are the consequence of common inflammation, they are
comparatively under the most favourable circumstances for recovery; but they are much
more frequently the consequence of an inflammation depending on a particular constitution, viz. what is called scrofulous; and
in this case they are almost always fatal.

Tubercles

There is no morbid appearance so common in the lungs as that of tubercles. These
consist of rounded firm white bodies, interspersed through their substance. They are
I believe formed in the cellular structure,
which connects the air cells of the lungs together, and are not a morbid affection of
glands, as has been frequently imagined.
There is no glandular structure in the cellular connecting membrane of the lungs;
and on the inside of the branches of the tra-

chea, where there are follicles, tubercles have
never been seen. They are at first very small,
being not larger than the heads of very small
pins, and in this case are frequently accumulated in small clusters. The smaller tubercles of a cluster probably grow together, and
form one larger tubercle. The most ordinary size of tubercles is about that of a garden pea, but they are subject in this respect
to much variety. They adhere pretty closely to the substance of the lungs, and have no
peculiar covering or capsule. When cut into, they are found to consist of a white
smooth substance, having great firmness, and
often contain in part a thick curdly pus.
When a tubercle is almost entirely changed
into pus, it appears like a white capsule in
which the pus is lodged. When several tubercles of considerable size are grown together, so as to form a pretty large tuberculated
mass, pus is very generally found upon cutting into it. The pus is frequently thick and
curdly, but when in considerable quantity
it is thinner, and resembles very much the

pus from a common sore. In cutting into
the substance of the lungs, a number of abscesses is sometimes found from pretty large
tubercles having advanced to a state of suppuration. In the interstices between these
tubercles, the lungs are frequently of a
harder, firmer texture, with the cells in a
great measure obliterated. The texture of
the lungs on many occasions, however,
round the boundaries of an abscess, is perfectly natural.

I have sometimes seen a number of small
abscesses interspersed through the lungs,
each of which was not larger than a pea.
The pus in these is rather thicker than what
arises from common inflammation, and resembles scrofulous pus It is probable that
these abscesses have been produced by a
number of small scattered tubercles taking
on the process of suppuration. The lungs
immediately surrounding these abscesses are
often of a perfectly healthy structure, none
of the cells being closed up by adhesions.

When tubercles are converted into abscesses, it forms one of the most destructive diseases in this island, viz. pthisis pulmonalis. Tubercles are sometimes found in the lungs of children at a very early age, viz. two or three years old, but they most frequently occur before the completion of the growth. They are apt likewise to be formed at rather an advanced age.

In cutting into the lungs, a considerable portion of their structure sometimes appears to be changed into a whitish soft matter, somewhat intermediate between a solid and a fluid, like a scrofulous gland just beginning to suppurate This appearance I believe is produced by scrofulous matter being deposited in the cellular substance of a certain portion of the lungs, and advancing towards suppuration It seems to be the same matter with that of the tubercle, but only diffused uniformly over a considerable portion of the lungs, while the tubercle is circumscribed.

I have seen another sort of tubercle in the lungs, which I believe to be very rare It consists of a soft tumour, formed of a light brown, smooth substance. This is not contained in any proper capsule, but adheres immediately to the common structure of the lungs. In cutting through several of these tumours I did not find any of them in a state of suppuration. They were commonly as large as a gooseberry, and were chiefly placed upon the surface of the lungs; some, however, were scattered through their substance, of a smaller size. These are very different in their appearance from the common tubercle last described, and are the effect of a diseased process, which probably is very imperfectly known.

In opening into the chest, it is not unusual to find that the lungs do not collapse, but that they fill up the cavity completely on each side of the heart. When examined, their cells appear full of air, so that there is seen upon the surface a prodigious number of small white vesicles. The branches of the trachea are at the same time much filled with a mucous fluid. This is not uncommonly the case in persons who have laboured for some considerable time with difficulty of breathing, but without any symptoms of inflammation; such persons would appear to die from want of a supply of atmospheric air sufficient to produce the proper change in the blood which is necessary for its useful circulation through the body.

The lungs are sometimes, although I believe very rarely, formed into pretty large cells, so as to resemble somewhat the lungs of an amphibious animal. These cells, in the only instance which I have seen of this disease, were most of them of the size of a common garden pea, and some few were so large as to be able to contain a small gooseberry. They were surrounded by a fine transparent capsule, and were so numerous as to occupy more than one half of the portion of the lung which I saw. The only specimen of this sort of disease which I am acquainted with, is in the collection of Mr. Cruikshank; and the person in whom it was found, had been very long subject to difficulty of breathing.

The lungs are sometimes converted into a solid substance very much resembling the liver. It has nearly the same solidity, and the same general appearance. When examined more minutely, the air cells appear to be filled with a brownish solid matter. It is very obvious, that as this process spreads over the lungs, respiration must become more difficult ; there will be less room for the admission of air, in order to produce that change upon the blood which is necessary for the preservation of life, and this circumstance will produce a more frequent respiration, in order to endeavour to remedy the deficiency.

Part of the lungs is occasionally converted into a bony substance, but this is a very rare disease The small vessels disposed through the substance of the lungs under such circumstances separate bony matter from the blood. In the only instance which I have known of this complaint, the process would appear to have been rapid. There was great difficulty of breathing before the person died, but this difficulty had only begun for a very few weeks. Each lung was undergoing the same process, which had made considerable advancement. In the particular case to which I allude there had been a very strong disposition to form bone in the constitution. A very large bony tumour had been formed round one of the knees of this person ; and very soon after the knee and leg were removed by amputation, the difficulty of breathing began, which was occasioned by a part of the lungs being converted into bone. Here was a transference of this peculiar disease from an external to an internal part, similar to the translation of gout or rheumatism.

I have also seen a tumour as large as an orange, attached to the lungs on one side by a loose membranous connection, and in some degree compressing them ; this tumour consisted of a yellowish, porous substance, which neither resembled the structure of what is commonly understood to be a schirrous or scrofulous tumour, but had an appearance somewhat peculiar to itself. It was probably the effect of a morbid action with which we are very little acquainted.

Earthy concretions have occasionally been found in the lungs, although it is a rare appearance of disease. These are often small, but sometimes form pretty large masses.* Even a considerable portion of the lungs has been known to be changed into an earthy substance.†

Hydatids are also sometimes formed in the lungs, and are many of them brought up by coughing. Of their nature I propose to treat particularly afterwards.

* Vid. Morgagni, Epist XVII Art. 19. Epist. XV. Art. 25
† Vid. Morgagni, Epist. XXII Art 15.

CHAP. V.

Diseased Appearances in the Posterior Mediastinum.

By the posterior mediastinum, is meant that space which lies between the laminæ of the pleura, that pass from the root of the lungs to each side of the spine. The space is of considerable size, and contains a portion of the trachea arteria, of the œsophagus, of the thoracic duct, of the descending aorta, and the vena azygos, besides some absorbent glands.

Diseased Appearances of the Trachea.

The inner membrane of the trachea is not uncommonly inflamed to a greater or less degree. In this state it is crowded with

minute florid vessels, which give it a general appearance of vascularity. When
there is no inflammation, it appears a white
pulpy membrane, but there are rarely to be
seen any red vessels ramifying through it.
While the inner membrane is inflamed, the
secretion from its glands is very much increased, and therefore its cavity is found a
good deal filled with a mucous fluid ; even
pus is sometimes formed, and both fluids are
mixed with globules of air. This is probably the situation of the trachea in a very
violent catarrh, and also in some cases
where there are scrofulous abscesses of the
lungs, attended with hoarseness, and a sense
of soreness along the trachea.

When the inner membrane of the trachea
is inflamed, it is sometimes lined with a
layer of a yellowish pulpy matter. This
does not adhere very firmly to the inner
membrane, but may be easily separated.
It extends from the upper part of the cavity of the larynx, into the small branches
of the trachea, which are distributed through

the substance of the lungs. There is at the same time a good deal of mucus in the trachea, and its branches, together with a mixture of pus. This is the appearance of the inside of the trachea, in patients who have died from the croup.

Polypus.

The trachea and its branches are sometimes lined with a layer of a yellowish matter, forming a sort of tube, which is applied to the inner surface loosely. It has not occurred to me to see any instance of it in the dead bodies which I have examined, but I have seen several examples of it in preparations. The inner membrane of the trachea seems to be perfectly natural, and the layer of adventitious membrane resembles exactly the coagulable lymph, that is thrown out in other parts of the body; I have therefore no doubt of its being that substance. Since this disease (which is called polypus) lasts for a long time, and is not attended with symptoms of inflammation, it appears probable, that the vessels of the inner membrane of the trachea possess a power of separating the coagulable lymph from the blood, and that this disease consists in a peculiar action of these vessels.

The trachea has been said to be sometimes filled with a solid substance of the same kind with what we have described; but in the instances which I have seen, it has been tubular; and I believe this to be by much the most common appearance.

The trachea I have seen narrowed in diameter for two or three inches, thickened in its substance, and the inner membrane has been raised into a number of little hard tubercles. This state of the trachea was accompanied with a schirrous affection of some absorbent glands, which closely adhered to it; and it appeared to me, that the disease in the glands had spread so as to affect the trachea

The cartilaginous rings of the trachea

occasionally become ossified, although this is not a very frequent appearance. The change is so natural from cartilage into bone, that we should be led to expect it more commonly. When the ossification is inconsiderable, the function of the trachea will hardly be affected, but where the rings are entirely ossified, the flexibility of the trachea must be much lessened, and its cavity will not admit of being so much contracted as in the healthy state, by the action of the muscular fibres, which form a part of its structure. The consequence of this must be, that the mucus which is occasionally accumulated will not be so readily expelled by coughing, and the air will not be thrown out in so small a column, nor with so much momentum.

The trachea is no doubt liable to be destroyed in part by ulceration, from causes acting immediately upon itself, but in the instances which I have seen, the ulceration has been connected with ulceration of the œsophagus. As the œsophagus is more liable to this disease, it is probable that in such cases the ulceration has begun in the œsophagus, and spread to the trachea.

Diseased Appearances of the Œsophagus.

The œsophagus is frequently lined with a layer of the coagulable lymph, which is continued from the cavity of the mouth.

This, it is said, sometimes extends over the whole intestinal canal, but I should believe this appearance to be extremely rare, and it commonly terminates at the lower end of the œsophagus. The inner membrane of the mouth is much more vascular than in its natural state, shewing an intense dark red colour, but in examinations after death the appearance of greater vascularity is sometimes little observable in the œsophagus. This disease is known under the name of apthæ, and is much more often to be observed in the living than the dead body. Portions of the coagulable lymph are thrown off, and other portions formed several times in the progress of the disease.

The œsophagus is liable to stricture, produced by the contraction of its muscular fibres at some particular part. This disease is I think most common in women whose constitutions are delicate, and much subject to nervous influence. When such a disease is examined in the dead body, the œsophagus is found to be more or less contracted in some part of it, and it feels harder than usual, as all muscles do in a contracted state. There is no appearance of diseased structure usually combined with it. I can suppose, however, that this contraction might lay the foundation of a permanent, and even a fatal disease. The muscular fibres of the œsophagus might so press on the inner membrane, as to excite inflammation in it, which might advance to suppuration, and would most probably terminate fatally.

I once saw a very unusual stricture of the œsophagus. It consisted in its inner membrane being puckered together, so as to form a narrowness of the canal at a particular part. The canal at that part, was so narrow, as hardly to allow a common garden pea to pass. There was no appearance, however, of diseased structure in the inner membrane which was so contracted, and the muscular part of the œsophagus surrounding it was perfectly sound. I know that this disease was very slow in its progress, for the person in whom it took place had been for many years affected with a difficulty of swallowing, and could only swallow substances of extremely small size.

The most common appearance of disease in the œsophagus, is that of an ulcer in its cavity. Ulcers of the œsophagus are sometimes of a common nature, but most frequently they are attended with a schirrous affection When ulcers of the œsophagus arise from common inflammation, the structure of the œsophagus immediately surrounding the ulcer is little thickened, and there is the appearance of the usual erosion in ulcers When the ulcer is of a schirrous nature, the œsophagus in the neighbourhood

is very much thickened, and is very hard in
its texture. When this texture is examined,
it either consists of an hard, uniform, fleshy
substance, or this is a little intersected by
a membranous appearance, or it is gristly.
Under such circumstances, the canal of the
œsophagus is always more or less narrowed,
and in some cases is almost wholly obliterated   It is worthy of remark, that these ulcers happen most frequently, either immediately under the pharynx, or near the cardia.

Any substance capable of irritating the
inner membrane of the œsophagus, by having
sharp hard projections, will no doubt be more
likely to affect the œsophagus, where it first
enters into it.   In an œsophagus, therefore,
predisposed to schirrus, such an accident
may prove an exciting cause, and the disease
will more frequently take place at its upper end.   At the cardia too, there is a peculiar arrangement of the muscular fibres,
which are capable of acting in some degree
like a sphincter, and which probably produce on many occasions a narrowness of

canal there. This will render the œsophagus at the cardia more liable to be injured
by the passage of any hard substance, and
may ultimately lay the foundation of a schirrous ulcer. This is the account which the
late Dr. Hunter used to give of the frequent
situation of ulcers at the upper and lower
extremities of the œsophagus, and seems to
have great weight. It happens, however,
most commonly that ulcers of the œsophagus arise spontaneously, or in other words,
from causes within itself which we cannot
ascertain. When an ulcer takes place at the
upper end of the œsophagus, it is apt to
spread into the substance of the thyroid
gland. In this case the gland becomes hard,
enlarged, and ulcerated.

A portion of the œsophagus has been observed by some anatomists to be converted
into cartilage, and to have its diameter at
that part very much diminished in size.*
This was, perhaps, only a strong example of
the gristly texture which we have above described, or it may have been a change into a

* Vid. Bonet, Tom 2 p 32.

substance like common cartilage. In this case it is a very uncommon appearance of disease.

I have seen an instance of a fungus arising on the inside of the œsophagus, which is to be considered as a rare disease. When cut into, it appeared to have a fibrous structure, disposed in some measure at right angles to the inner membrane upon which it was formed, and was ulcerated on its surface.

The pharynx, at its lower extremity, has been known to be dilated into a pouch of considerable size, which passed behind the œsophagus. This may be supposed to be very rare, but there is an instance of it preserved in Dr. Hunter's collection. The pouch in this case began to be formed in consequence of a cherry-stone having rested there for some time, which had made a kind of bed for itself. It remained in that situation for three days, and then was brought up by a violent fit of coughing. A part of the food always rested afterwards in the cavity made by the cherry-stone, by

F

which it was gradually enlarged. At length, in the course of about five years, the cavity was enlarged into a bag of a considerable size, sufficient to contain several ounces of fluid. This bag passed down a good way behind the œsophagus, and the œsophagus necessarily acquired a valvular communication with it. In proportion as the bag enlarged, this valvular communication would become more and more complete, till at length every kind of food must have rested in the bag, and could not pass into the œsophagus In this way the person was destroyed The lower end of the pharynx is, perhaps, the only part of the canal where such an accident could happen The pharynx is not contracted gradually, so as to lose itself insensibly in the œsophagus, but contracts itself rather suddenly at the lower end Hence a little recess is formed, in which an extraneous body may occasionally rest. This is necessarily at the posterior part, so that if the recess should be enlarged into a cavity, it must pass behind the œsophagus

The particulars of this singular case have been published in the Medical Observations *

The Descending Aorta.

There is hardly any other disease of the descending aorta within the posterior mediastinum, than aneurism. This consists in the aorta being a good deal enlarged beyond its natural size, in its coats being irregularly thickened, and more readily divisible into layers There are also frequently deposited behind the inner membrane little thin laminæ of bony matter. This appearance of disease, has been formerly explained more particularly. It is rare that this part of the aorta becomes aneurismal, unless there be a general aneurismal affection over the arterial system.

The Vena Azygos.

The vena azygos is very seldom diseased.

* See the Medical Observations, Vol 3, p. 85.

I have seen it however varicose, and very much enlarged. This change in it took place from particular circumstances. A considerable portion of the vena cava inferior had become obliterated; in consequence of this, the usual vena azygos, together with an uncommon one on the left side, were the only channels through which the blood could return by a circuitous route to the heart; they were therefore necessarily, from the impetus of the blood, much enlarged in size, and for the same reason likewise varicose. This case I have more particularly described in the Medical and Chirurgical Transactions.*

The vena azygos has been known to be ruptured, when very much distended with blood.† Such a case has not come under my own observation, and I should believe it to be very uncommon.

* See p 125, &c.
† Vid Morgagni, Epist. XXVI. Art. 29.

The Thoracic Duct.

The thoracic duct is also subject to very few diseases. I have never seen any other, except that of its being very much enlarged beyond its natural size, and varicose.

In the instance to which I allude, it was very nearly as large as the natural size of the subclavian vein, but nothing could be detected in the neighbouring parts, capable of accounting for this appearance. There was no obstruction at the entrance of the thoracic duct into the venal system, which might naturally have been expected. This diseased appearance of the thoracic duct has already been taken notice of in Mr. Cruikshank's Treatise on the Absorbent System.*

The thoracic duct has been known to be obstructed by an earthy matter deposited in its cavity.† It does not necessarily happen, when the thoracic duct is at some part

---

* See second edition, p. 207; and it is represented in an engraving, plate V.

† Vid. Lieutaud, Tom. 2, p. 93.

obstructed that chyle is prevented from entering into the system of blood vessels. The thoracic duct not unfrequently sends off one or more considerable branches, which unite again with the principal trunk. If under such circumstances an obstruction should take place in a part of the principal trunk, between the origin and the termination of those branches, no bad effect would follow; one or more of those branches would become enlarged and convey the chyle in its full quantity to the blood

The thoracic duct has also been known to be ruptured, although this is exceedingly rare.

Absorbent Glands

The absorbent glands in the posterior mediastinum, as well as in every other part of the body, are liable to several diseases. The most common morbid affection is scrofula In this case they are frequently a good deal enlarged, and feel somewhat

softer to the touch than in their healthy
structure. When cut into, however, they
frequently exhibit very much the natural
appearance; but it is more common to find
that some of them contain a white, soft,
cheesy matter, mixed with a thick pus;
this is the most decided mark of scrofulous
affection. When the absorbent glands in
this situation are very much enlarged, they
necessarily produce some difficulty of
breathing, both by pressing on the lungs
and the trachea. They might produce also
some difficulty of swallowing.

I have seen the absorbent glands in the
neighbourhood of the trachea affected with
schirrus, although it is a rare disease in them.
They were much enlarged, and very hard
to the touch. When cut into, they exhibited a hard brownish structure, somewhat
intersected by white firm membrane, so as
to resemble exactly what is called schirrus
in other parts of the body. The trachea in
contact with these glands was also affected.
In this case the thyroid gland was schir-

rous, and it is probable that the disease spread from the thyroid to the absorbent glands, and so to the trachea.

The absorbent glands near the trachea are sometimes converted into a bony or earthy matter, from a peculiar secretory action in their blood vessels; and I think that this disease is more common in the absorbent glands at the root of the trachea, than in any other part of the body. These glands when so diseased, by pressing against the trachea or œsophagus, occasionally produce ulcers in them.

The Anterior Mediastinum.

By the anterior mediastinum is meant the space inclosed between the laminæ of the pleura, which pass from the sternum to the pericardium; it contains little else than cellular membrane, with perhaps a small portion of fat; and in the younger subject, the thymus gland.

It is seldom found with any diseased appearance in it. Abscesses are occasionally formed there, but rarely. Water too is sometimes found in the cells of its cellular membrane. I have also seen air accumulated in these cells.

Fat is occasionally deposited in the mediastinum in considerable quantity. When the quantity is very large, it has been known to disturb a good deal the functions both of the heart and lungs. The thymus gland I have known to be much enlarged beyond its natural size, and to have a schirrous hardness.

CHAPTER VI.

—————

Diseased Appearances within the Cavity of the Abdomen.

Ascites.

ASCITES, or dropsy of the cavity of the abdomen, is a very frequent disease, and is not
confined to any sex or age I have seen
several instances of it in children under ten
years old, but it is much more common at
the middle, and the more advanced periods
of life It is also more common in the
male than the female sex When water
is accumulated in a very considerable quantity in the cavity of the abdomen, the su-
perficial veins of the belly are generally a
good deal distended with blood; this most
probably arises from the pressure of the
water upon the deeper seated veins; it is
however sometimes hardly observable even

when the accumulation of the water is very considerable. The skin at the navel is also often protruded, yielding easily to pressure, but this is not universally the case. On many occasions the protrusion can hardly be seen, when the water is accumulated in large quantity. In opening into the cavity of the abdomen, there is to be seen a larger or less quantity of an aqueous fluid, generally of a brownish colour, but its colour varies according to circumstances. When there is a schirrous liver accompanying the dropsy, the water is commonly of a yellowish or greenish colour. This arises from a mixture of the bile with the water, and under such circumstances there is almost always a jaundiced colour of skin. I have seen the water in ascites of a chocolate or coffee colour; but this appearance is rare. In the case to which I allude, the water was thicker than that of ascites usually is, but it had the common properties, as far as could be known from the application of heat or of acids   When there are none of the viscera of the abdomen diseased, the water in ascites resembles the serum of the blood in its colour, as well as in its other properties.

While water is accumulated in the cavity of the abdomen, the intestinal canal is frequently found to be somewhat in a contracted state ; but often too this is not observable. In many cases of ascites the liver is diseased, being hard and tuberculated, as we shall explain particularly when treating of the diseases of the liver. In some cases too, the spleen has been found to be enlarged and hard.

The ascites is not necessarily connected with the accumulation of water any where else in the body, but it frequently happens that it is accompanied with the accumulation of water in the chest, and under the skin, particularly of the lower extremities.

Inflammation of the Peritonæum.

The peritonæum is not uncommonly inflamed, although it is by no means so liable to this disease as the pleura. There is a cause of inflammation in it peculiar to women, arising from the state of the womb after parturition; but there is also a variety of causes producing it, which are equally applicable to both sexes, so that it is frequently found in men, and also in women who have not been pregnant.

When inflammation has taken place in the peritonæum, there are several appearances to be taken notice of in opening the body. The peritonæum is thicker than in its natural state, more pulpy, and less transparent; and it is crowded with a number of very small vessels, carrying a florid blood. When a portion of the inflamed peritonæum is separated from the abdominal muscles, there is commonly no appearance whatever of the inflammation having spread

into the muscles, but where the peritonæum covers the intestinal canal, the inflammation is sometimes found to have pe-
netrated not only into the muscular coat
of the intestines, but even into the villous
membrane. The reason of this difference
probably is, that the peritonæum is less connected with the abdominal muscles than
with the intestinal canal, so that the inflammation is more easily confined in the one
case than in the other.

The inflammation of the peritonæum is
sometimes slight and partial , at other times,
is great and universal. When it is slight, and
affects that part of the peritonæum which is
connected with the intestinal canal, it often
forms broad bands of inflammation which
run along the course of the intestines,
and are bounded by the contact of the different portions of the intestines among
themselves   In this case, the coats of the
intestine are not thicker than usual, the inflammation being slight and confined to the
peritonæum itself   Where the inflamma-

tion is great, the intestines are much thicker, and more massy. This evidently arises from the greater accumulation of blood in the small blood vessels, as well as from the extravasation of fluids into the substance of the intestines, in consequence of the strong inflammatory action of the vessels. The mesentery and mesocolon are much thicker than in their natural state, and there is also a remarkable change in the omentum. It is frequently as thick as a person's hand, and lies as a circumscribed mass along the great curviture of the stomach. The principal cause of this change in these parts is the extravasation of coagulable lymph into the cellular membrane between the laminæ of the peritonæum which form them.

In many places there is thrown out a layer of a yellowish pulpy matter, gluing different portions of the viscera together. This is sometimes a thin layer, at other times is of considerable thickness: and it appears to be the coagulable lymph of the blood. The layer of the coagulable lymph

is often found to extend beyond the immediate surface which is inflamed. This arises
from the coagulable lymph being thrown
out from the vessels in a fluid state, and
therefore need not be limited by the boundaries of the inflamed surface when it becomes solid. There is also a considerable
quantity of a brownish fluid in the cavity
of the abdomen, resembling the serum,
which is mixed with small shreds of the coagulable lymph, and sometimes with pus,
giving it a turbid appearance. The quantity of the coagulable lymph, and of the
fluid, is sometimes large, in proportion to
the degree of the inflammation. Air is frequently too found accumulated in the stomach and the intestinal canal, which had
been formed in the progress of the disease.
At other times this air is wanting.

Adhesions in the Cavity of the Abdomen.

When there has been inflammation of the
peritonæum either generally or partially,

sufficient to have thrown out coagulable lymph, and the patient has survived the disease, the coagulable lymph is changed into a fine transparent membrane, which is the membrane of adhesions. The time which is occupied in the change of the coagulable lymph into the membrane of adhesions, is not very long, for I have had several opportunities of tracing the gradual progress of the change from the one into the other, while the inflammation appeared to have been recent. This membrane consists of a cellular substance, similar to the general cellular membrane of the body, and has a moderate share of vascularity. It does not naturally shew many vessels large enough to admit the red globules of the blood, but it shews its vascularity upon slight degrees of inflammation, or by using the fine injection. This membrane is capable of elongating gradually by the motion of the viscera upon themselves, so as ultimately to be attended with very little inconvenience. I have very often had an opportunity of observing these adhesions, either joining all the viscera of the abdomen more or less together, or joining some particular viscera to each other.

I have observed also pus formed in an inflamed state of the peritonæum; but I have never seen this membrane mortified independent of the mortification of some of the viscera.

I have several times had an opportunity of observing a white soft granulated matter, adhering universally behind the peritonæum In some places it formed a mass of considerable thickness; in others, it was scattered in single small masses. In one case I recollect it formed a substance as thick as my hand, between the peritonæum and the abdominal muscles, while it was scattered in small separate portions in the mesentery and the peritonæum, covering the intestinal canal. The omentum I have sometimes seen changed into a cake of this substance The matter itself appeared to me to be scrofulous, for it resembled exactly the

structure of a scrofulous absorbent gland
before pus is actually formed. I am not at
all certain how far this appearance of disease should have been classed along with
those of the peritonæum: it does not take
place (at least in the cases which I have
seen) in the peritonæum itself, but behind it,
yet at the same time adhering to it. It
appears, however, upon the whole, to be
placed here with more propriety than it
could have been any where else.

I have also seen some small cancerous
tumours growing from the peritonæum.
These were extremely hard, of a white colour, and resembled exactly in their structure
the cancerous masses which are formed in
the stomach. What puts the appearance I
allude to beyond doubt, is, that in the same
body I found a cancerous tumour of the
stomach. The cancerous tumours of the
peritonæum were not at all connected with
this other, but were in that part of the membrane which lines the recti abdominis muscles,

nearly opposite to the region of the stomach.

Hydatids have occasionally been found to occupy a portion, or even the whole, of the cavity of the abdomen. In such cases many of them are connected with the viscera, which were probably the basis of their formation, of which the chief are the liver, and the spleen. This appearance of disease is very uncommon.

Air has been occasionally said to be accumulated in the cavity of the abdomen, while little or none is contained in the intestines.* This I believe to be a very rare occurrence. Air is not unfrequently found accumulated in considerable quantity in the intestinal canal, while there is none at all in the cavity of the abdomen.

* Vid Lieutaud, Tom 1, p. 432

CHAP. VII.

Diseased Appearances of the Stomach.

Inflammation.

It sometimes happens, although not very frequently, (unless poisons have been swallowed) that inflammation takes place in the stomach, so as to spread over a very considerable portion of its inner membrane, or perhaps the whole of it. It is much more common, however, for inflammation to occupy a smaller portion of the stomach. In such cases too, the inflammation is generally not very violent. The stomach upon the outside, at the inflamed part, shews a greater number of small vessels than usual, but frequently not much crowded. In opening into the stomach, it is found to be a little thicker at the inflamed part, the inner membrane is very red from the number of small florid vessels, and there are frequently spots of extravasated blood. It does not often occur that a common inflammation of the stomach proceeds to form pus, or to terminate in gangrene.

When arsenic has been swallowed, (which is the poison most frequently taken) the stomach is affected with a most intense degree of inflammation. Its substance becomes thicker, and in opening into its cavity there is a very great degree of redness in the inner membrane, arising partly from the very great number of minute vessels, and partly from extravasated blood Portions of the inner membrane are sometimes destroyed, from the violent action that has taken place in consequence of the immediate application of the poison. I have also seen a thin layer of the coagulable lymph thrown out upon a portion of the inner surface of the stomach. Most commonly too some part of the arsenic is to be seen in the form of a white powder, lying upon different portions of the inner membrane.

In opening the bodies of persons who have died from hydrophobia, the inner membrane of the stomach is frequently found inflamed at the cardia, and its great end. This inflammation, however, is generally inconsiderable, is, I believe, never very great, and in some instances has been said to be wanting.

Ulcers of the Stomach.

Opportunities occasionally offer themselves of observing ulcers of the stomach. These sometimes resemble common ulcers in any other part of the body, but frequently they have a peculiar appearance. Many of them are hardly surrounded with any inflammation, nor have they irregular eroded edges as ulcers have generally, nor is there any particular diseased alteration in the structure of the stomach in the neighbourhood. They appear very much as if some little time before a part had been cut out from the

stomach with a knife, and the edges had
healed, so as to present an uniform smooth
boundary round the excavation which had
been made. These ulcers sometimes destroy only a portion of the coats of the stomach at some one part, and at other times
destroy them entirely. When a portion
of the coats is destroyed entirely, there is
sometimes a thin appearance of the stomach
surrounding the hole, which has a smooth
surface, and depends on the progress of the
ulceration   At other times, the stomach is
a little thickened surrounding the hole; and
at other times still, it seems to have the
common natural structure.

Schirrus and Cancer of the Stomach.

This affection of the stomach is not very
uncommon towards an advanced period of
life, and, I think, is more frequently met with
in men than in women. This, perhaps, arises
from the greater intemperance in the one
sex, than in the other. It cannot, however,

be produced entirely by intemperance;
there must be added a considerable predis-
position of the parts towards this disease.
Hence, when there is no previous disposition, the stomach does not become affected
with this disease, whatever be the intemperance. When, however, there is this previous disposition, there is reason to think that
it is encouraged and brought forwards by
this mode of living.

Schirrus sometimes extends over almost
every part of the stomach, but most commonly it attacks one part. The part
which is affected with schirrus has sometimes no very distinct limit between it and
the sound structure of the stomach, but
most commonly the limit is very well
marked. When schirrus attacks a portion
of the stomach only, it is generally towards
the pylorus. The principal reason of this
probably is, that there is more of glandular
structure in that part of the stomach than
in any other; and it would appear that
glandular parts of the body are more liable

to be affected with schirrus, than parts of the body generally.

When the whole stomach, or a portion of it, is schirrous, it is much thicker than usual, as well as much harder. When the diseased part is cut into, the original structure of the stomach is frequently marked with sufficient distinctness, but very much altered from the natural appearance. The peritonæal covering of the stomach is many times thicker than it ought to be, and has almost a gristly hardness. The muscular part is also very much thickened, and is intersected by frequent pretty strong membraneus septa These membranous septa are, probably, nothing else than the cellular membrane intervening between the fasciculi of the muscular fibres, thickened from disease. The inner membrane is also extremely thick and hard, and not unfrequently somewhat tuberculated towards the cavity of the stomach.

It very frequently happens that this thickened mass is ulcerated upon its surface, and then a stomach is said to be cancerous. Sometimes the inner membrane of the stomach throws out a process which terminates in a great many smaller processes, and produces what has been commonly called a fungous appearance.

It also happens that the stomach at some part loses entirely all vestige of the natural structure, and is changed into a very hard mass, of a whitish or brownish colour, with some appearance of membrane intersecting it; or it is converted into a gristly substance, like cartilage somewhat softened. The absorbent glands in the neighbourhood are at the same time commonly enlarged, and have a very hard white structure.

I have seen several instances of a schirrous tumour being formed in the stomach about the size of a walnut, while every other part of it was healthy. This tumour has most frequently a small depression near the middle of its surface, and appears a little radiated in its structure. While this tumour remains free from irritation, the functions of the stomach are probably very little affected by it ; when, however, it is irritated, it must occasion very considerable disorder in the functions of the stomach, and perhaps lay the foundation of a fatal disease.

A part of the stomach is occasionally formed into a pouch by mechanical means, although very rarely. I have seen one instance of a pouch being so formed, in which five halfpence had been lodged. The coats of the stomach were thinner at that part, but were not inflamed or ulcerated. The halfpence had remained there for some considerable time, forming a pouch by their pressure, but had not irritated the stomach in such a manner as to produce inflammation or ulceration.

The orifice of the stomach may be almost, or perhaps entirely, shut up by a permanent contraction of its muscular fibres, either at the cardia or the pylorus. It is much more likely, however, to occur most frequently at the pylorus, from natural circumstances. there is both less opposition to prevent the

contraction at this orifice of the stomach
than at the cardia, and there is also belonging to it a stronger and more direct circular
muscular power.   A less contraction too, at
the pylorus, will produce an obstruction in
the canal, than at the cardia.   I have seen
one instance of this contraction at the pylorus, which, even there, is a very rare disease.   The contraction was so great as
hardly to admit a common goose quill to
pass from the stomach into the duodenum,
and it had prevented a number of plum
stones from passing, which were therefore
detained in the stomach.

The stomach is sometimes found so contracted through the whole of its extent as
not to be larger than a portion of the small
intestine ; at other times, it is enlarged to
much more than its ordinary size   Neither
of these appearances are to be considered as
arising from disease.   They depend entirely on the muscular fibres of the stomach
being in a state of contraction or relaxa-
tion, at the time of death.   It happens, I

think, more frequently that the stomach is dilated than contracted.

The stomach is very commonly found, in a dead body, flaccid and almost empty, but not unfrequently it is found more or less distended with air: this air may have been formed after death, but it is often formed during life. When this is the case, we may suppose it to be produced by a new chemical arrangement in the contents of the stomach, but, I believe, it more frequently happens that air is separated from the blood in the blood vessels of the stomach, and poured by the small exhalants into its cavity. This has been more particularly taken notice of by Mr. Hunter, in his Essay upon Digestion,* and by myself, in a paper which is published in the Medical and Chirurgical Transactions. †

In looking upon the coats of the stomach at its great end, a small portion of them

* See Mr Hunter's Observations on certain parts of the animal economy, p 164

† See case of emphysema, p. 202

there appears frequently to be thinner, more transparent, and feels somewhat more pulpy than is usual, but those appearances are seldom very strongly marked. They arise from the action of the gastric juice resting on that part of the stomach in greater quantity than any where else, and dissolving a small portion of its coats. This is therefore not to be considered as the consequence of a disease, but as a natural effect arising from the action of the gastric juice, and the state of the stomach after death. When the gastric juice has been in considerable quantity, and of an active nature, the stomach has been dissolved quite through its substance at the great end, and its contents have been effused into the general cavity of the abdomen. In such cases the neighbouring viscera are also partially dissolved. The instances, however, of so powerful a solution are rare, and have almost only occurred in persons who while in good health had died suddenly from accident. The true explanation of these appearances was first given by Mr. Hunter, and published, at the request of Sir John Pringle, in the Philosophical Transactions.*

Tumours, consisting of a suetty substance, have been sometimes found in the stomach, but they are to be considered as a very rare appearance of disease. Ruysch relates that he has seen a tumour from the stomach of a man which contained hair, together with some dentes molares; and this he has preserved in his collection. †

Calculi with different appearances have been described as being occasionally found in the stomach. They have never come under my own observation, and are to be reckoned very uncommon. ‡

Papillæ and pustules, somewhat resembling the small-pox, have also been described as being formed on the inner membrane of the stomach, but these are exceedingly rare. ‖

* See Philosoph Transact Vol 62, p. 447.

† Vid Ruysch, Tom. 2 Adversar Anatomicor Decad. Tert

‡ Vid Lieutaud, Tom 1, p 17

‖ Vid Lieutaud, Tom 1, ⸬ 23

Even true small-pox pustules have been said to be formed in the stomach of persons who have died from this disease.* In later dissections, however, this appearance has not been observed, so that, at least, it must be considered as very uncommon.

* Vid. Lieutaud, Tom. 1, p. 371.

H

[98]

CHAP. VIII.

Diseased Appearances in the Intestines.

Inflammation.

THE intestinal canal is subject to inflammation from a variety of causes, and therefore it is very usual to observe its effects after death   When a portion of intestine is inflamed, there is spread upon its outer surface a number of small vessels, many of which are carrying a florid blood.   When the intestine is cut into, so as to exhibit its inner membrane, it appears highly vascular, from the small vessels of the villi being loaded with blood, and there are frequently to be seen a few spots of blood extravasated. In inflammation of the intestines, the peritonæum is often very little, or not at all affected When the inflammation, however, is very great, the peritonæum is also inflamed, and covered with a layer of coagulable lymph.

I have likewise seen, in violent inflammation, scattered portions of coagulable lymph thrown out upon the surface of the villous membrane. The intestine is at the same time much more thick and massy than in a healthy state, and its colour is sometimes very dark, from a large quantity of black extravasated blood. This state of an intestine has often been mistaken for mortification.

It very commonly happens that inflammation of the intestines advances to suppuration and ulceration. Ulceration, however, does not appear to be so common in the small as in the great intestines. When it takes place either in the one or the other intestine, it is attended with considerable variety in its appearance · the edges of the ulcer have sometimes considerable thickness, at other times, they are not thicker than the healthy structure of the intestine; the edges and general cavity of an ulcer are sometimes ragged, and at other times they are smooth, as if a portion had been cut out from the intestine with a knife. Sometimes, through a considerable length of the intes-

tine (especially the great one) the inner
membrane hangs in tattered shreds, occasioned by the great ravage of the ulceration. I have also seen a considerable portion of the intestine completely stripped of
its inner membrane, from the extent of this
process, and its muscular coat appeared as
distinct as if it had been very carefully dissected. In the follicular glands, which are
gathered together in little oval groups, I
think I have seen ulceration more frequently than in the other parts of the intestine

When ulceration advances very actively,
it sometimes eats through the coats of an intestine entirely. When this is the case, a
portion of the contents of the intestine occasionally passes into the general cavity of
the abdomen, producing there inflammation.
This, however, does not very often happen,
most commonly that portion of the gut
where the ulcer is situated, adheres by inflammation to some other portion, or to a
neighbouring viscus, and a communication
is formed between the one and the other
I have seen communications formed in this

manner between the rectum and the bladder
in a male, and between the rectum and the
vagina in a female. I have even seen a
communication formed between the kidney
and a portion of the intestine from this
cause, by which the pus produced in the
kidney was evacuated through the intestine. Those communications are the means
of preserving life (although in a very uncomfortable state,) for a much longer time
than it could be, were the matter to pass into the general cavity of the belly. It would
there produce peritonæal inflammation,
which would very soon destroy.

Inflammation of the intestines sometimes,
although rarely, advances to mortification.
When this is the case, the mortified part is
of a dark livid colour, and has lost its tenacity, it is in this state very easily torn
through, or the fingers will pass through it
as through a rotten pear. The want of the
natural tenacity, when attended with the
other circumstances which we have mentioned, is the only sure criterion of a part

being mortified, in examinations after death.
A portion of intestine may be of a very
dark colour, and yet may not be mortified.
This darkness of colour may be occasioned
by a large quantity of extravasated blood
thrown out during a high degree of inflammation, where the principle of life is main-
tained in full vigour. Thus we see blood
effused into the cellular membrane under
the skin producing a very dark appearance,
yet the parts are all alive. It has often
happened too, that a very dark portion of
intestine has been returned in the operation
for the bubonocele, and yet the parts have
recovered their natural functions. This
could never have happened if the black portion of the intestine had really been mortified Under such circumstances, the mortified part would have separated from the
living, and the function of the gut must have
been destroyed When a portion of gut has
been for some time mortified, there is formed a considerable quantity of air, which is
accumulated in its cavity This is a part

of the natural process which takes place in
all dead animal substances.

Intus Susceptio.

This is a disease which is not very uncommon, and which is frequently fatal. It consists in a portion of gut passing for some
length within another portion, and there
also enters along with it a part of the mesentery. The portion of gut which is received into the other, is found generally in
a contracted state, and is sometimes of considerable length It usually happens that
an upper portion of intestine falls into a
lower; but the contrary likewise occurs, although rarely Intus susceptio may take
place in any part of the intestinal canal,
but it happens most frequently in the small
intestine, and also where the ilium terminates in the colon. In this last situation, it
appears to me to happen more frequently
than any where else. This, perhaps, depends on the great disproportion in bulk

between these two portions of intestine. In opening into the bodies, particularly of infants, an intus susceptio is not unfrequently found, which had been attended with no mischief: the parts appear perfectly free from inflammation, and they would probably have been easily disentangled from each other by their natural peristaltic motion. At other times, however, violent inflammation takes place, the parts are thickened and glued together by adhesions, and the passage of the intestines is obstructed. This is the fatal state of the disease.

Ruptures.

A portion of the viscera of the abdomen frequently passes out of that cavity, being lodged in a bag of elongated peritonæum, and this disease is called a rupture. It happens most commonly from some sudden and violent concussion of the body, where the weaker parts of the parietes of the abdomen give way; it is a more frequent disease too, I think, among fat than lean people: this depends on the increased size of the viscera, which therefore press with more force against the sides of the abdomen. There is hardly any viscus which has not, at some time or other, been found in the sack of a rupture, but most frequently it is either a portion of the omentum, or of the intestine. The bag formed by the elongated peritonæum may be thrust out almost at any part of the belly, but this happens more frequently at the ring of the external oblique muscle, under Paupart's ligament, and at the navel: it also, sometimes, takes place at other parts of the abdomen. The most usual situation of a rupture in the male, is at the ring of the external oblique muscle; and this arises probably from the larger size of that opening in the male, than in the female. The most usual situation of a rupture in the female is either under Paupart's ligament, or at the navel. The reason of the frequency of the first situation, is the particular shape of the pelvis

in the female, by which there is a larger
empty space under Paupart's ligament, than
in the male, so that the viscera here are
less firmly supported. The reason why
the second situation of a rupture occurs
often in the female, is, probably, frequent
child-bearing During pregnancy, at its
advanced period, the navel opens, or gives
way, and where pregnancies have been frequent, it pr bably never recovers its original strength.

The viscus which is most commonly found
in the sack of a rupture, is the omentum.
This, perhaps, arises from its being a loose
mass, not tied down to any particular situation, and therefore it readily passes into any
cavity which communicates with the abdomen When it has once fallen down, it has
no means of pulling itself out, like a portion
of intestine, which is another reason why
it is so often found in a rupture. When it
has remained long in any sack, it forms a
pretty compact mass, sometimes having no
connection with, but at other times adher-

ing to the inner surface of the sack. There is frequently no inflammation produced in the omentum while in this situation, but occasionally violent inflammation takes place, which may even advance to mortification.

A portion of gut is very often lodged in the sack of a rupture, either by itself, or along with a portion of the omentum. The portion of gut is sometimes very small, but at other times it is very considerable. Very often the functions of the intestines go on properly in this situation, but occasionally violent inflammation is produced, interrupting their function, and often terminating fatally. This inflammation is produced by the pressure of the narrowest part of the sack against the gut, viz. that part of the sack which immediately passes out of the cavity of the abdomen. This inflammation exhibits the different appearances, upon dissection, which we have so often explained. The gut too, is frequently found mortified: this is shewn by its dark colour, by its want of proper tenacity, and by the air which is formed. When the inflammation of the gut in a sack has not been very violent, and has receded, it frequently leaves adhesions behind it, connecting the gut with the inner surface of the sack It is perhaps possible too, that adhesions may be formed by long close contact, without inflammation.

When the sack of a rupture has not been of long standing, it consists of a thin, firm, white, opaque, membrane; this is an elongation of the peritonæum, somewhat thickened by pressure. When the sack has been of long standing, it is often very thick, and evidently consists of a number of layers The sack upon the inside has a very smooth surface, and the membrane which forms this surface can be readily traced into the peritonæum, lining the cavity of the abdomen; the outer surface of the sack is more rough and coarse in its texture: the sack, where it passes out of the cavity of the abdomen, has frequently a narrow

neck, or aperture, and is distended below
into a bag of considerable size. At other
times, the communication between the sack
and the cavity of the abdomen, is by a larger
opening. Under these circumstances there
is less danger of inflammation being produced by pressure against the gut.

In bubonocele, or that species of rupture which takes place at the ring of the
external oblique muscle, the sack is usually
quite distinct from the sack of the tunica
vaginalis testis. At other times, there is no
separation between them, but the contents
of the rupture are immediately in contact
with the body of the testicle: this kind of
rupture is called the hernia congenita. It
was formerly supposed, when it happened,
to arise from a portion of the sack of the
rupture and of the tunica vaginalis giving
way, so that the contents of the rupture fell
into the cavity of the tunica vaginalis testis,
and came in contact with the testicle.
Upon a little reflection, it might have been
seen that this could hardly take place; but

the true account of this appearance was not known till it was explained by Dr. Hunter. Baron Haller discovered, that till about the eighth month the testicles do not descend into the scrotum, but are situated in the cavity of the abdomen under the kidneys. When they descend into the scrotum, the peritonæum which covers them is necessarily drawn down along with them through the ring of the external oblique muscle; it then forms a bag, whose upper extremity communicates with the cavity of the abdomen Baron Haller had also observed, that in infants a portion of intestine sometimes falls down into this bag after the testicle, or along with it, producing what he called the hernia congenita. The communication between the bag and the abdomen is commonly soon closed, for it is not open at birth It appears, however, if it is prevented from closing at the usual time, that it does not close afterwards, but remains open through life Hence, if any portion of an intestine, or of the omentum falls into the elongated sack of the peritonæum, it must be in contact with the testicle. When Dr. Hunter became acquainted with the observations of Baron Haller upon the descent of the testicles, he saw at once that the species of rupture sometimes to be met with in adults, where a portion of intestine or omentum is in contact with the testicle, might be easily explained. His explanation corresponded with what we have just given, and has been universally adopted by anatomists and surgeons.

Schirrus and Cancer of the Intestines.

Schirrus is a disease which takes place much more commonly in the great than in the small intestines, but the latter are occasionally affected by it. I have seen both a schirrous tumour, and a cancerous ulcer in the duodenum. In the great intestine at an advanced period of life, schirrus is not uncommon, it is not equally liable to affect every portion of this intestine, but is to be found much more frequently at the sigmoid flexure of the colon, or in the rectum, than any where else; the reason of this it is, perhaps, difficult to determine. There is certainly more of glandular structure in the inner membrane of the great intestine towards its lower extremity, than in any other part of it, and I think that this sort of structure has a greater tendency to be affected with schirrus, than the ordinary structures of the body: the gut, too, is narrower at the sigmoid flexure than at any other part, and therefore must be more liable to be injured by the passage of hard bodies; these, by their irritation, may excite the disease of schirrus in a part which was pre-disposed to it. What we have now said, however, is merely conjectural.

The schirrus sometimes extends over a considerable length of the gut, viz. several inches; but generally it is more circumscribed. When it is affected with schirrus, it exhibits the same appearances of structure which were described when speaking of schirrus

of the stomach. The peritonæal, muscular,
and internal coats are much thicker and harder
than in a natural state. The muscular too
is subdivided by membranous septa, and the
internal coat is sometimes formed into hard
irregular folds. It often happens that the
surface of the inner membrane is ulcerated,
producing cancer. When schirrus affects
the gut, the passage at that part is always narrowed, and sometimes so much so
as to be almost entirely obliterated. The
obliteration, or stricture, would sometimes
appear to be greater than in proportion to
the thickness of the sides of the diseased
gut this, most probably, depends upon
the contraction of the muscular fibres of the
gut, which, although diseased, have not altogether lost their natural action. Where
the passage is very much obstructed, the
gut is much enlarged immediately above
the obstruction, from the accumulation of
contents in that part of the intestine.
While this disease is going on in a portion
of the intestine, adhesions are formed be-

tween it and the neighbouring viscera, and the ulceration sometimes spreads from the one to the other.

The inner membrane of the great intestine I have seen a good deal thickened, and formed into small irregular tubercles, some of which were of a white, and others of a yellowish colour ; the peritonæal and muscular coats were also thicker and harder than in a natural state This is not a frequent appearance of disease, but it has sometimes been found to take place in very severe dysenteries, such as in that which has been described by the late Sir John Pringle.*

I have also seen the internal membrane of the great intestine formed into broad thick folds, in which a considerable quantity of blood was accumulated ; these folds were perfectly independent of the state of the contraction in the muscular coat, and were very different in their appearance from

* See Pringle's Diseases of the Army, p. 246.

the irregular puckering which is often seen
in the inner membrane of the great intestine. When these folds were examined,
they were found to consist of an accumulation only of cellular membrane, lying behind the inner coat of the gut   What was
the effect of this diseased structure in the
living body, I had no opportunity of learn-
ing.

Upon the inner surface of the great intestine, about two inches above the anus, little processes sometimes grow from the internal membrane: they generally surround the gut at short distances from each
other, so as to form a sort of circle.

Piles, and fistulæ in ano, are diseases
which are extremely common, but which
hardly ever become an object of examination after death, they have therefore not
been so commonly introduced into accounts
of morbid appearances as others which
much more rarely occur   Piles are soft
tumours commonly situated round the verge
of the anus, sometimes of a regularly

bulbous, at other times of an irregular form. They are covered with a very tender skin, which partly consists of the fine skin immediately round the anus on the outside, and partly of the inner membrane of the gut. The tumours are generally entire, but they have occasionally small openings through which a considerable quantity of blood is sometimes poured; they consist of the extremities of the branches of the mesaraica minor vein, much enlarged from the accumulation of blood.

The same sort of tumours are also frequently found within the cavity of the rectum, forming what have been called, the internal piles. Piles are a much more frequent disease in persons who are advanced in life, than in those who are young. They arise from repeated, and long continued impediments to the return of the blood by the branches of the mesaraica minor vein, and there has been much more opportunity for these impediments to act in old, than in young persons. They are

also more common in women than in men.
This may arise from several causes: the
uterus during pregnancy must occasion a
great impediment to the return of the blood
from the rectum ; this is so much the case,
that women who have been frequently
pregnant seldom escape piles. Women too
are more apt to allow of an accumulation
of the proper contents of the rectum, than
men, and this will produce some impediment to the return of the blood from this
part. It may perhaps be added, that the
greater weakness of the original formation
in women, than in men, may render the
former more liable to this disease than the
latter.

Fistulæ in ano, are narrow canals at the
lower end of the rectum, with a smooth internal surface, with callous edges, and
having the power of secreting pus.* A disease of this sort may consist of one canal,

* Mr Hunter has observed, in his Lectures on Surgery,
that fistulæ have a smooth internal surface, like a secreting
surface, as, for instance, the urethra.

opening by a very small aperture externally, at the side of the anus; or this
canal may be divided into several branches
When this last is the case, the disease is
more serious, as it requires for its cure a
more difficult, tedious, and painful operation. The canal, besides opening externally, has very commonly a small opening
into the gut itself; and sometimes there is
a small opening into the gut, without
there being any externally on the side of the
anus It is much more common, however,
that there should be an external opening
of the canal only; or, that there should both
be an external opening, and another into
the gut

It is a species of monstrous formation,
not very uncommon, that the rectum does
not terminate in the anus, but in a cul-de-
sac, without reaching the external surface.
Sometimes the extremity of the gut lies
immediately behind the skin, which is there
thinner, and shews where the anus ought
to have been placed Under these circum-

stances, it is easy to make an artificial anus. It happens often, however, that the rectum terminates more than an inch behind the skin, and then a remedy by an operation is much more difficult, and uncertain.

I have also seen the rectum terminate in the bladder, from an original error in the formation, so that there was no other external opening to the rectum than by the urethra : this was in a child at birth ; the mal-formation was of such a kind, as neither to admit of a remedy by art, nor to allow of life being continued. The rectum has also been known to terminate in the vagina, from a defect in the original formation ; but this is very uncommon.

Worms

Worms are formed in the intestines of man, as well as of many other classes of animals, but not so frequently in the former as in the latter. In most quadrupeds and fishes it is extremely common to find a number of worms upon opening their intestines.

The worms which are found in the human subject, may be reduced to three general classes, viz the lumbricus teres; tænia, and ascaris.

Lumbricus Teres

The lumbricus teres, or round worm, is much more commonly found in the intestines of children, than in those of persons full grown, or advanced in life: it is very usually met with in the first, but rarely in the two last. The lumbricus teres has been often confounded with the common earth worm, to which it bears a general resemblance, although it is really very different. By most practitioners, indeed, at present, there is known to be a difference, yet it is not very well understood in what this difference consists The two species of worms, if attentively examined, will be found to differ a good deal from each other in their external appearance The lumbricus teres is more pointed at both extremities, than the common earth worm; the mouth of the lumbricus teres consists of three rounded projections, with an intermediate cavity. The mouth of the earth worm consists of a small longitudinal fissure, situated on the under surface of a small rounded head. Upon the under surface too of the worm there is a large semilunar fold of skin, into which the head retreats, or out of which it is elongated, which is entirely wanting in the lumbricus teres. The anus of the lumbricus teres opens upon the under surface of the worm, a little way from its posterior extremity, by a transverse curved fissure ; the anus of the earth worm opens by an oval aperture at the very extremity of the worm. The outer covering or skin in the lumbricus teres is less fleshy, and less strongly marked by transverse rugæ, than in the earth worm. In the latter there is often to be seen a broad white band, surrounding the body of the worm ; but in the lumbricus teres, this is entirely wanting. On each side of the lumbricus teres there is a longitudinal line very well marked ; in the earth worm there are three longitudinal lines upon the upper half of its surface, but these are faintly marked, so as to be hardly observable. The lumbricus teres has nothing corresponding to feet; whereas the earth worm has on its under surface, and towards its posterior extremity, a double row of processes on each side, very sensible both to the eye, and the finger, which manifestly serve the purposes of feet in the locomotion of the animal.

The internal structure of both animals is also extremely different. In the lumbricus teres, there is an intestinal canal, nearly uniform and smooth in its appearance, which passes from one extremity of the worm to the other ,* in the earth worm, there is a large and complex stomach, consisting of three cavities; and the intestinal canal in the latter is likewise larger, and more formed into sacculi, than the former. The parts subservient to generation are very different in both: in the lumbricus teres there is a distinction of sex, the parts of

* Near the head of the lumbricus teres, the canal is narrower than it is any where else, and also somewhat distinct in its limits, which may be considered as the œsophagus.

generation being different in the male and in
the female ; in the common earth worm the
organs of generation are the same of each
individual, as this animal is hermaphrodite.
The appearance too of the organs of generation, is extremely different at first sight
in the one species of animal, and the other :
There is an oval mass situated at the anterior extremity of the earth worm, resembling a good deal the medullary matter of
the brain ; in the lumbricus teres this substance is wanting * These are the greater
differences between the one species of animal and the other, which are obvious upon
a very moderate attention to each Many
other differences would, no doubt, be found
by a person who might choose to prosecute
their anatomy minutely.

Tænia.

The tænia, or tapeworm, is rarely found
in the intestines of the inhabitants of this

---

* What this substance is I do not know, and I have only
mentioned its resemblance to the medullary matter of the
brain, in order to give a clearer description of it.

country, but is very common in those of some countries on the continent, particularly Switzerland. It consists of a great many distinct portions, which are connected together so as to put on a jointed appearance; these joints are commonly of a very white colour, but are occasionally brownish, which depends on a fluid of this colour that is found in their vessels. The worm is usually very long, extending often many yards, and seldom passes entire from the bowels. This circumstance has prevented the extremities of the tænia from being often seen.

The head of a tænia is somewhat of a square form, with a narrowed projection forwards ; in the middle of this projecting part, there is a distinct circular aperture, around which is a single, or a double row of curved sharp processes. At the square edge of the head, there are situated four round projecting apertures, at equal distances from each other : this head is placed upon a narrow jointed portion of the worm, of considerable length, and which gradually spreads itself into the broader joints, of which the body of the worm is composed.

The body of the tænia, which is most commonly found in the human subject, consists of thin, flat, pretty long joints, on one edge of which there is a projection, with a very obvious aperture. In the same worm some of these joints appear considerably longer than others ; this probably depends on one joint being contracted, while another is relaxed The apertures which we have just mentioned are generally placed on the alternate edges of the contiguous joints : but this is not uniformly the case; they are sometimes placed on the same edges of two, or even several contiguous joints. When these joints are examined attentively, there are frequently seen, in each of them, vessels filled with a brownish fluid, and disposed in an arborescent form. Around the edges of each joint, there is also a distinct serpentine canal.* The last joint of a tænia resembles very much a

This, as well as the vessels disposed in an arborescent

common joint rounded off at its extremity, and without any aperture. The description which I have given, is chiefly taken from what I have seen myself, and corresponds, I believe, with what is most common. There are differences, however, in tæniæ described by authors, chiefly with regard to the number and situation of the oscula of the joints, so as to distinguish them into different species; but they are all formed upon one general plan.

Ascaris.

The ascaris is a very small worm, which is often found at the lower end of the rectum in children, and even more frequently in adults than is commonly imagined. It is white in its colour, and about half an inch in length; it is a little narrowed at the extremity where its head is placed, and at the

form, is very distinctly seen injected in some preparations which have been made, and given to me by an ingenious young surgeon, Mr Carlisle

other extremity it terminates in a long, very
fine, transparent process. These worms
are more or less surrounded with mucus,
and this is probably secreted in greater
quantity by the glands in the inner membrane of the rectum, from the irritation occasioned by the worms.

There is nothing in the economy of animals more obscure than the origin of intestinal worms; were they found to live in
situations out of the bodies of living animals, one might readily suppose that their
ovula were taken into the body along with
the food and drink, and there gradually
evolved into animals. This, however, is
not the case; they do not seem capable of
living for any length of time in any situation, except within a living animal body,
which appears to be the proper place for
their growth and residence. We might
therefore be led to another supposition, viz.
that intestinal worms are really formed
from the matter contained in the intestines,

which previously had no regular organization ; but this idea is widely different from
all analogy in the production of animals,
where there has been any satisfactory opportunity of examining this production.
The origin therefore of such animals is a
subject of much obscurity, nor do I pretend
at all to throw any light upon it. When
the whole evidence, however, in support of
the one and the other opinion is compared
together, I own, that the grounds for be-
lieving that in some orders of animals equi-
vocal generation takes place, appear stronger
than those for a contrary opinion.

It is not unusual to find air accumulated
in the intestinal canal, in greater or less
quantity ; this air is sometimes accompanied with a slight inflammation of the
peritonæum, and at other times it is not.
In such cases the blood vessels, creeping
upon the intestines, are frequently filled
with air, but not uncommonly they are
without it. Air is often let loose into the

intestines after death by putrefaction; but that which we wish particularly to consider here, has been formed during life.

There are only two ways in which we can well conceive air to be formed in the intestines· the one is, some new arrangement in the contents of the intestines, by which air is extricated: the other is, the formation of air in the blood vessels of the intestines by a process similar to secretion, and which air is afterwards poured out by the extremities of the exhalant arteries into the cavity of the intestines. That the blood vessels of an animal body have this power there can be no doubt; and I own I am inclined to think that this is a very frequent mode by which air is accumulated in the intestines. This air probably differs somewhat at different times: in several trials which I have made, it never shewed signs of containing any proportion of inflammable air, but always a very sensible proportion of fixed air. It requires, however, to be examined by some person well.

K

acquainted with chemical experiments, in order that its ingredients may be exactly ascertained.

These are the more common appearances of diseased, or preternatural structure in the intestines; but I have likewise had an opportunity of observing others, which are of rarer occurrence. In one or two instances, I have seen a sort of bony matter thrown out upon the surface of the inner membrane of the gut: I have even seen an adhesion between two portions of intestine, converted into bone. It would appear, that almost every part of the body is endued with a power of taking on this process. It may not improperly be considered, as a natural process misplaced. An adhesion being once formed, has the same power (as far as we know) of running into different processes, as the cellular membrane, which makes a part of the original structure It may therefore form bone, as readily as cellular membrane, or some other membranes of the body, which have a resemblance to the membrane of adhesions, as the pleura, and the peritonæum.

I have seen one of the valvulæ conniventes much larger than usual, and passing round on the inside of the jejunum, like a broad ring. The canal of the gut was necessarily much narrowed at this ring, but no mischief had arisen from it. This mal-formation, however, might have laid the foundation of fatal mischief. Some substance too large to pass, might have rested on the ring, and produced there inflammation, ulceration, and ultimately death.

Calculous matter has sometimes been known to be accumulated in some part of the cavity of the intestinal canal, especially the great intestine; but this has not come under my own observation, and, at least in the human subject, is a very rare occurrence.*

Small-pox pustules have been said to be sometimes formed in the intestines of persons who have died from this disease.† How

* Vid Lieutaud, Tom 1, p 77, 78,
† Vid. Lieutaud, Tom 1, p. 371.

far this may have occasionally taken place, I will not pretend to say, but late dissections, upon the best authority, have not confirmed this fact.

Diseased Appearances of the Mesentery.

The mesentery is often found in a state of inflammation, although I believe this hardly ever takes place, unless when the peritonæum generally is inflamed. When the mesentery is inflamed, it becomes much thicker, and more massy, than in its natural state; the large blood vessels, which pass between its laminæ and the absorbent glands, are also very much obscured. These different appearances depend upon the quantity of the coagulable lymph which is thrown out, during the inflammatory action The peritonæum which forms the laminæ of the mesentery is crowded with small blood vessels, and is covered more or less with a layer of the coagulable lymph A small quantity of pus is sometimes found

on the surface of an inflamed mesentery,
and even abscesses have been observed between its laminæ ; but this last appearance
is very rare.

It very seldom happens, that the mesentery is found gangrenous, unless different
portions of the intestinal canal be found in
the same state. It has not occurred to me,
at least, to see an instance of this sort.
When the intestines are mortified, portions
of the mesentery are generally found in the
same condition. The appearances exhibited in mortification are the same when
it affects the mesentery, as any other part,
and they have been already explained.

The absorbent glands of the mesentery,
are frequently found to be scrofulous, and
this is more apt to take place in children,
than at a more advanced age. When affected with this disease, the glands exhibit
different appearances, according to its progress : they are enlarged in their size, and
are softer to the touch, than in a natural
state When cut into, they sometimes shew

very much the natural structure; but more frequently they are changed, in part, into a white, soft, curdly matter, and this is not uncommonly mixed with pus. When the absorbent glands of the mesentery are universally affected with scrofula, and very much enlarged in their size, the abdomen is very tumid, and the face and extremities appear a good deal emaciated.

When a portion of the intestinal canal becomes cancerous, some of the absorbent glands in the mesentery generally become affected with the same disease: this is in consequence of the matter of cancer being conveyed to those glands by absorbent vessels The glands become enlarged in size, and are changed into hard masses of a schirrous, or cancerous texture.

The absorbent glands of the mesentery are sometimes found filled with an earthy, or bony matter; but this is to be considered as a rare occurrence.* The absorbent glands

* Vid. Med. Transactions, Vol. I, p. 361.

at the root of the lungs, are more liable to be affected with this disease.

Hydatids have also been occasionally found adhering to the mesentery.

Tumours, likewise, consisting of a fatty matter, have been seen attached to the mesentery; but these I believe to be very uncommon.

CHAP. IX.

Diseased Appearances of the Liver.

Inflammation of the Membrane of the Liver.

THE external membrane of the liver is not uncommonly found in a state of inflammation

This may either take place when the peritonæum generally over the cavity of the abdomen is inflamed, or the inflammation may be confined to the membrane of the liver itself. When it is confined to the membrane of the liver, I think it is not frequently extended over the whole of it, but more commonly takes place in that part which covers the anterior, or convex part of the liver I have also seen inflammation, or at least its effects, not unfrequently on that side of the liver, which is in contact with the stomach and the duodenum.

When inflammation takes place in the membrane of the liver, it exhibits exactly the same appearances, which have been described when speaking of the inflammation of the peritonæum, of which it is a part. It is crowded with a great number of very minute vessels, which carry a florid blood, and is thicker than natural. There is also thrown out upon its surface, a layer of coagulable lymph ; this layer is thicker on some occasions than others, and often glues the liver, more or less completely to the neighbouring parts. There is at the same time thrown out, some quantity of serous fluid.

Adhesions.

It is more common to see adhesions formed, which are the consequence of a previous inflammation in the membrane of the liver, than to see the membrane in an actual

state of inflammation. These adhesions
are formed from the coagulable lymph of
the blood, which undergoes a gradual progress of change, as we have formerly described. They consist very commonly of a
thin, transparent membrane, which joins
the surface of the liver to the neighbouring parts. This junction may either be
general, over one extended surface of the
liver, or it may consist of a number of processes of adhesion : the adhesion is sometimes by a membrane of considerable
length ; at other times, the adhesion is
very close, the surface of the liver being
immediately applied to the neighbouring
parts. The surface of the liver, where
these adhesions are most commonly found,
is the anterior, by which it is joined to
the peritonæum lining the muscles at
the upper part of the cavity of the abdomen.

When an abscess is formed in the substance of the liver, and points externally,
these adhesions are of great use in prevent-

ing the pus from escaping into the general cavity of the abdomen. Adhesions are also frequently found connecting the posterior surface of the liver to the stomach, and the duodenum ; and these may also be useful in abscesses of the liver, near its posterior surface, by preventing the matter from passing into the general cavity of the abdomen, and conducting it either into the stomach, or the upper part of the intestinal canal.

Inflammation of the Substance of the Liver.

It does not often happen, at least in this country, that the substance of the liver is actually found in a state of inflammation. Where its membrane is inflamed, the substance is sometimes inflamed which lies immediately under it ; but it rarely happens that the general mass of the liver is inflamed In warmer countries, the substance of the liver is much more liable to inflammation than in Great Britain. When the liver is generally inflamed through its substance, it is a good deal enlarged in size, and of a deep purple colour.* It is also harder to the touch, than in its healthy state. Its outer membrane is sometimes affected by the inflammation, and at other times is not. It is frequently accompanied with a jaundiced colour of skin, arising from the bile not getting readily into the ductus communis choledochus, on account of the pressure of the inflamed liver on the pori biliarii When this inflammation has continued for some time, abscesses are formed, and then the active state of the inflammation very much subsides. These abscesses are sometimes of large size, so as even to contain

---

* May not the purple colour arise from the accumulation of blood in the branches of the vena portarum ?

As this vein most probably performs the office of an artery in the liver, is it not probable, that its small branches take on the same actions as the small branches of an artery during inflammation

some pints of pus. Sometimes the whole of the liver is almost converted·into a bag containing pus. When inflammations of the liver have been of considerable stand-ing, they are not uncommonly attended with ascites, and the water is of a yellow, or green colour, being tinged by the bile.

The liver has sometimes been said to have been in a state of mortification * This however occurs very rarely, and has never fallen under my own observation.

Common Tubercle of the Liver.

One of the most common diseases in the liver (and perhaps the most common, ex-cept the adhesions which we have lately described) is the formation of tubercles in its substance. This disease is hardly ever met with in a very young person, but fre-quently takes place in persons of middle or advanced age. it is likewise more com-mon in men than women. This would

* Vid. Morgagni, Epist XXXIV. Art 25

seem to depend upon the habit of drinking being more common in the one sex than in the other, for this disease is most frequently found in hard drinkers, although we cannot see any necessary connection between that mode of life and this particular disease in the liver It happens, however, very commonly, that we can see little connection between cause and effect in changes which are going on in every other part of the body.

The tubercles which are formed in this disease occupy generally the whole mass of the liver, are placed very near each other, and are of a rounded shape. They give an appearance every where of irregularity to its surface. When cut into, they are found to consist of a brownish or yellowish white solid matter. They are sometimes of a very small size, so as not to be larger than the heads of large pins; but most frequently they are as large as a small hazel nut, and many of them are sometimes larger. When the liver is thus tuberculated, it feels

much harder to the touch than natural, and
not uncommonly its lower edge is bent a
little forwards. Its size, however, is generally not larger than in a healthy state, and
I think it is sometimes smaller. If a section
of the liver be made in this state, its vessels
seem to have a smaller diameter than they
have naturally. It very frequently happens
that in this state the liver is of a yellow colour, arising from the bile accumulated in its
substance; and there is also water in the cavity of the abdomen, which is yellow, from
the mixture of bile. The gall-bladder is generally much contracted, and of a white colour, from its being empty. The bile, from
the pressure of the hard liver upon the pori
biliarii, does not reach the ductus hepaticus,
and therefore cannot pass into the gall-
bladder. The colour of the skin in such cases
is jaundiced, and it remains permanently
so, as it depends on a state of liver not liable
to change. This is the common appearance of what is generally called a schirrous
liver: but there are other hard tubercles

formed in it, which resemble more the structure of schirrus in other parts of the body.

Large white Tubercle of the Liver.

Hard white masses are sometimes formed
in the liver, of a considerable size. They are
often found as large as a chesnut, but I have
seen them both a good deal larger and
smaller than this size. They are to be found
near the surface of the liver in greater number, than near the middle of its substance
two or three frequently lie contiguous to
each other, with a considerable portion of
the liver, in a healthy state, interposed between them and a cluster of similar tubercles. They consist of a very firm, uniform,
opaque, white substance, and generally
somewhat depressed, or hollow, upon their
outer surface. The liver in this disease is
frequently a good deal enlarged beyond its
natural size

These tubercles appear to be first formed
round the blood vessels of the liver, as is

seen in making sections of a liver in this
state. While the liver is under such circumstances of disease, there is sometimes
water in the cavity of the abdomen, and at
other times none; the liver is sometimes
tinged in its colour, from the accumulation
of bile, and at other times the colour of its
substance between the tubercles is perfectly
natural.

The kind of tubercle which we have now
described, is much more rare than the other,
and resembles much more the ordinary appearance of schirrus in other parts of the
body Were I to determine, therefore, simply
from structure, I should consider the large
white tubercle as the true schirrus of the
liver; and the other may, perhaps, be some
peculiar disease of this viscus, which is
found as difficult of cure as the true schirrus What I have now said is merely conjectural, and intended to excite a greater attention to this subject

Soft brown Tubercles of the Liver.

I have also seen in the liver a number of soft tumours, about the size of a walnut they were principally situated at the surface of the liver, and consisted of a smooth, soft, brownish matter. This is a very rare appearance of disease, and its real nature is probably not thoroughly known. Such tumours might perhaps be called scrofulous, but there is no strong evidence in support of this opinion; and there is certainly no resemblance between this sort of tumour and either a scrofulous tubercle of the lungs, or a scrofulous absorbent gland. It would be worth while, as such appearances occur, to examine them particularly, so that at length the nature of the disease may be ascertained This inquiry will be much assisted by an accurate knowledge of the symptoms, and of the general tendency of the constitution in the living body.

Scrofulous Tubercles of the Liver.

Tubercles are occasionally found in the liver which resemble exactly the tubercles of the lungs, but this is a very rare appearance of disease. They have the same size, the same structure, and the same feeling to the touch In the only instance which I have seen of this disease, the tubercles were generally dispersed through the substance of the liver at pretty regular distances, and did not render the surface of the liver irregular, as in the common sort of tubercle.

I have likewise seen the liver much more flaccid in its substance than is natural, with reddish tumours, of considerable size, interspersed through it, which contained a thick sort of pus I am inclined to consider this liver as scrofulous, because it was found in a person whose general constitution had strong indications of scrofula, and where there were found many scrofulous absorbent glands on examining the body

L 2

Liver very soft in its Substance.

The liver is not unusually found much more flaccid in its substance than natural, without any other appearance of disease. It feels upon such occasions nearly as soft as the spleen, and is commonly of a leaden colour. This change must arise from a process which takes place through its whole substance, and seems to be what Mr. Hunter has called the interstitial absorption. By this process is meant, where the absorbents remove insensibly small ingredient parts out of the general mass of any structure in an animal body without ulceration. This state of liver is very rarely, if ever, found in a very young person, and is most common in persons who are advanced in life.

Liver very hard in its Substance.

There is a very contrary state of the liver, not at all unusual, viz. where it is much harder than natural, and when cut into, exhibits no peculiar mode of structure. Upon the surface of these livers, there is not uncommonly a thready appearance of membrane, disposed somewhat in a radiated form, and the lower edge is bent a little forwards. This I believe to be the first step in the progress towards the formation of the common tuberculated liver. I have sometimes seen small tubercles formed upon a part of the surface of such a liver, which were exactly of the common sort. From this appearance, it is probable, that additional matter is deposited in the interstices, through the general mass of the liver, rendering it much harder, and that this matter, together with part of the ordinary structure of the liver, is converted into tubercles. What we have now said, however, is to be considered as entirely conjectural. This hardened state of liver is sometimes accompanied with a beginning ascites, and at other times is without it.

Hydatids.

There is no gland in the human body in which hydatids are so frequently found as the liver, except the kidneys, where they are still more common.* Hydatids of the liver are usually found in a cyst, which is frequently of considerable size, and is formed of very firm materials, so as to give to the touch almost the feeling of cartilage. This cyst, when cut into, is obviously laminated, and is much thicker in one liver than another. In some livers, it is not thicker than a shilling, and in others, it is near a quarter of an inch in thickness. The laminæ which compose it are formed of a white matter, and on the inside there is a lining of a pulpy substance, like the coagulable lymph. The cavity of the cyst I have seen subdivided by partitions of this

* although the hydatids of the liver, and the kidney, . . . the same name, yet there is reason to believe that . . . . from each other

pulpy substance. In a cyst may be found one hydatid, or a greater number of them. They lie loose in the cavity, swimming in a fluid; or some of them are attached to the side of the cyst. They consist of a round bag, which is composed of a white, semi-opaque, pulpy matter, and contain a fluid capable of coagulation. Although the common colour of hydatids be white, I have occasionally seen some of a light amber colour. The bag of the hydatid consists of two laminæ, and possesses a good deal of contractile power. On the inside of an hydatid, there are sometimes found smaller ones, which are commonly not larger than the heads of pins. These are attached to the larger hydatid, either at scattered irregular distances, or form small clusters they are also found floating in the liquor of the larger hydatids. Hydatids of the liver are often found loose and unconnected with each other; but at other times, they inclose each other in a series, like pill-boxes. The most common

situation of hydatids of the liver, is in its
substance, and inclosed in a cyst ; but they
are occasionally attached to the outer surface of the liver, hanging from it, and oc-
cupying more or less of the general cavity
of the abdomen.

The origin and real nature of these hydatids are not fully ascertained ; it is extremely probable, however, that they are a
sort of imperfect animals. There is no
doubt at all, that the hydatids in the livers
of sheep are animals: they have been often seen to move when taken out of the
liver, and put into warm water , and they
retain this power of motion, for a good
many hours after a sheep has been killed.
There is a great analogy, however, between
hydatids in the liver of a sheep, and in
that of the human subject. They are both
contained in strong cysts, and they both
consist of the same white pulpy matter.
There is undoubtedly some difference between them in simplicity of organization,
the hydatid in the human liver being a

simple uniform bag, and the hydatid in that of the sheep having a neck and mouth appended to the bag. This difference need be no considerable objection to the opinion above stated. Life may be conceived to be attached to the most simple form of organization. In proof of this, hydatids have been found in the brains of sheep, which resemble exactly those in the human liver, which have been seen to move, and therefore are certainly known to be animals. The hydatids of the human liver indeed, have not, as far as I know, been found to move when taken out of the body and put into warm water; were this to have happened, no uncertainty would remain. It is not difficult to see a good reason why there will hardly occur any proper opportunity of making this experiment. Hydatids are not very often found in the liver, because it is not a very frequent disease there; and the body is allowed to remain for so long a time after death before it is examined, that the hydatids must have lost their living principle, even if they were animals The probability of their being animals, however, is very strong; and it appears even more difficult to account for their production according to the common theory of generation, than for that of intestinal worms We do not get rid of the difficulty by asserting, that hydatids in the human liver are not living animals, because in sheep they are certainly such, where the difficulty of accounting for their production is precisely the same I have mentioned however already every thing I have to say upon this subject, when speaking of intestinal worms. If any person should wish to consider hydatids more minutely, he will find an excellent account of them published by Dr John Hunter in the Medical and Chirurgical Transactions *

Upon the inside of a cyst, exactly resembling that which contains hydatids, I have seen adhering a white, friable, earthy matter, what was its exact nature, I cannot

* See Medical and Chirurgical Transactions, p 34.

determine, but it was in some degree soluble in the marine acid.

Worms * have been said to be found in cysts of the liver, as well as in the biliary ducts Instances of this sort are extremely rare, and have not come under my own observation.

* Vid. Lieutaud, Tom. 1, p. 194.

CHAP. X.

Diseased Appearances in the Gall-bladder.

Inflammation of its Coats.

THE coats of the gall-bladder are very
rarely inflamed, independently of the inflammation of the membrane which covers the posterior surface of the liver.
When inflammation attacks this membrane,
it naturally spreads over the outer coat of
of the gall-bladder, which is a continuation
of it, and may affect the other coats of the
gall-bladder, if it should have arisen to a
violent degree. Inflammation, however,
of the outer coat of the gall-bladder will not
commonly be attended with inflammation
of the others, because it is not closely applied to them, there being interposed a
considerable quantity of cellular mem-

brane. The appearances of inflammation
in the coats of the gall-bladder, are exactly the same with what take place in the
inflammation of similar structures. These
we have already fully described, and shall
not here repeat them.

Adhesions.

It is a very common appearance, upon
dissection, to find the gall-bladder connected by adhesions, either to the small end of
the stomach, or the beginning of the duodenum These are the consequence of a
previous inflammation in the outer coat
of the gall-bladder, and resemble exactly
the adhesions which we have already described

It is rare that inflammation of the gall-
bladder advances to ulceration : the accumulation of gall-stones in it, very rarely
produces any effect of this kind. There is
but one instance of ulceration of the gall-
bladder which has fallen under my own

observation, and this is preserved in Dr. Hunter's collection.

Coats of the Gall-bladder schirrous.

I believe it to be very uncommon that the coats of the gall-bladder become schirrous. It has occurred to me, however, to observe one instance of it. The coats of the gall-bladder were in this case above a quarter of an inch in thickness, and studded with hard white tubercles, exactly similar to what we have described in the liver. indeed the liver to which this gall-bladder belonged was affected with the same disease. It is probable that the gall-bladder is scarcely ever affected with schirrus, unless it has previously taken place in the liver.

Coats of the Gall-bladder bony.

I have likewise seen the coats of the gall-bladder very much thickened, and converted in many parts into a sort of bony substance, but this is to be considered as a very rare appearance of disease.

Diseased State of Ducts.

There are two diseases in the excretory ducts of the liver and the gall-bladder which have come under my observation: the one is their obliteration, and the other their dilatation. The first is extremely rare, and the only instance which I have seen of it was in the ductus cysticus; the other is not uncommon The ductus hepaticus, ductus cysticus, and ductus communis choledochus, are sometimes dilated to an almost incredible size I have seen the ductus hepaticus and choledochus so much dilated as to be nearly an inch in transverse diameter. These dilatations of the biliary ducts hardly ever take place but from one cause, viz. the passage of gall-stones; and it is astonishing how large gall-stones sometimes are which have been known to pass into the duodenum. This ought to afford a good ground of comfort to persons who are labouring under this complaint.

It may not be improper to take notice here, that I have once seen an immediate communication, by a short canal, between the gall-bladder and the small end of the stomach. This lusus naturæ is very rare, and is probably attended with little inconvenience to the animal functions

Gall-stones.

It is not an uncommon appearance of disease in examining dead bodies, to find gall-stones, either in the gall-bladder, or in some of the biliary ducts. The gall-bladder is sometimes much enlarged in its size, and full of them In this case its coats are often a good deal thickened, and this probably arises chiefly from the efforts of the contractile power of the gall-bladder to expel them The number of stones accumulated in the gall-bladder is sometimes very great ; above a thousand have been taken out of one gall-bladder, which are preserved in Dr. Hunter's collection. When there is a solitary gall-stone in the gall-bladder, it is occasionally very large; I have known an instance of one which was fully the size of a hen's egg. When there is but one gall-stone either in the gall-bladder, or in the biliary ducts, it is generally of an oval shape; when there is a considerable number, they acquire, by rubbing upon each other, a great many sides and angles.

There is great variety in the external appearance of gall-stones with respect to colour· some are whitish, others are black; they are also of a yellowish, a greenish, a light brown, a dark brown, and a reddish-brown colour. These are the principal varieties in colour, but there are many other smaller differences which it would be very difficult to express in words. Gall-stones differ also very much in the smoothness of their surface, some being very smooth, and others a good deal tuberculated.

When cut or broken, gall-stones are com-

M

monly found to consist of concentric laminæ upon the out side, and in the centre of a
radiated texture. The laminated part bears
sometimes a large proportion to the other,
and at other times the contrary happens.
The laminated and radiated structures are
sometimes compact, and at other times consist of a loose matter. It likewise occasionally happens that both the laminated and the
radiated structures are very obscure, and the
gall-stone appears a good deal like an uniform solid mass The laminated part on
the outside very frequently consists of a different substance in appearance, from the
radiated structure in the centre ; and it is
not unusual to find the structure in the centre to consist of shining white crystalliza-
tions, which have a good deal the look of
spermaceti.

Gall-stones being very different both in
their outward appearance and their internal structure from each other, naturally lead
us to suppose that they may also differ in
their chemical properties. Upon this sub-

ject I can only speak very generally; but any trials which I have made incline me to this opinion. Very few gall-stones yield a bitter taste, which shews that they do not consist of inspissated bile; but in some I have found the taste intensely bitter. Almost all of them melt in the flame of a candle; but I have met with one sort, of a very black colour, which did not melt, but burnt exactly like a cinder.

All the gall-stones which I have examined dissolve in the nitrous acid. They are separated into a fine black powder when put into the vitriolic acid, especially if exposed to a sand heat. By the marine acid they are not acted upon at all in the common heat of the atmosphere, and are even but little affected by it when exposed to a sand heat for a considerable time.

Most of the gall-stones which I have examined are somewhat soluble in oil of turpentine, in the common heat of the atmosphere, but still not in a considerable degree; and one sort I have found to be in this heat altogether insoluble When put into this

M 2

oil, and exposed to a sand heat, they are much more readily acted upon. Some are converted into a kind of oil, which sinks to the bottom of the oil of turpentine; others are partly soluble, tinging the oil of turpentine of a brownish colour, and are partly separated into a powder.

Most gall-stones appear to be very little affected by spirit of wine in the common heat of the atmosphere, but are either partly or entirely soluble in it in a boiling heat.* Such are the general results from a good many trials of my own; but I speak upon this subject with very little confidence. It ought to be taken up by an able chemist, who is much in the habit of making experiments, and his experiments should extend to a great variety of gall-stones, which differ from each other in their appearance.

* When some biliary calculi are exposed to spirit of wine in a boiling state, white flaky crystals are soon formed upon its cooling. When they are exposed to spirit of wine in the common heat of the atmosphere, it is some weeks before crystals begin to be formed, and they appear to be more pointed in their shape than the former. These crystals were, I believe, first observed by M Poulletier de la Salle. See Elemens d'Histoire Naturelle et de Chimie, par M. de Fourcroy, Tom. 4, p. 354

Bile.

The bile in the gall-bladder is found to differ in different bodies; but this is too common to arise from disease, and must depend on natural circumstances. It is sometimes of a green, at other times of a brownish yellow, or a purer yellow colour. The brownish yellow colour is the most common. It is always more or less viscid, and the variety in this respect is considerable; in man it generally appears a good deal more viscid than in most other classes of animals. Upon one occasion, I have seen it as ropy as the mucus which is commonly coughed up from the trachea. In opening dead bodies, the bile is almost always found to have transuded in small quantity through the coats of the gall-bladder, so as to tinge the neighbouring parts, especially the small end of the stomach, and the beginning of the duodenum. This is to be considered as a natural effect, which has taken place after

death, and not as a diseased appearance.
The coats of the gall-bladder, in consequence of death, have lost that compactness
by which they were formerly able to con-
fine the bile ; it therefore transudes in small
quantity, and tinges the neighbouring parts

The gall-bladder is sometimes distended
with bile so as to be of nearly twice its
usual size; at other times, there is no bile
at all in its cavity, and under such circumstances it is white in its colour, and contracted into very small size.

It has been known to be distended to an
immense size, and to contain hydatids,* but
this state of it must be looked upon as extremely uncommon.

* See Medical Communications, Vol. 1, p. 101.

CHAP. XI.

Diseased Appearances of the Spleen.

Inflammation of the Coats of the Spleen.

THE coats of the spleen are liable to inflammation ; but this rarely takes place unless the peritonæum in the neighbourhood be also affected   The proper capsule of the spleen is so intimately connected with the peritonæum which is reflected over it, that it must necessarily partake of any inflammation affecting that portion of the membrane   When inflammation attacks the coats of the spleen, it exhibits exactly the same appearances which have been so often explained. They become much more crowded with vessels than in a natural state, are somewhat thicker, and throw out a layer of coagulable lymph.

Adhesions.

It is more common, however, to find adhesions formed between the spleen and the
neighbouring parts, than to find its coats
in an actual state of inflammation. These
adhesions consist of a white transparent
membrane of more or less firmness, and
generally connect more or less closely the
broad surface of the spleen to the dia-
phragm. They often connect too the
spleen to the great end of the stomach, and
a part of the transverse arch of the colon.

Inflammation of the Substance of the Spleen.

It is very rare to find the substance of
the spleen either in a state of inflammation
or suppuration; but such cases have occasionally been observed and related by authors * Instances also have been related
where the spleen has been observed to be

* Vid Lieutaud, Tom 1. p. 222

mortified,* but this I should believe to be even much more rare than the former.

The Spleen extremely soft.

There is an appearance of the spleen which is very common, and which perhaps is hardly considered as a disease, yet surely it is a very obvious deviation from its healthy structure. The appearance to which I allude, is an extreme softness of the spleen, so that when its capsule is broken (which under such circumstances is very tender), the substance of the spleen seems to be little else than a very soft, brownish-red mucus, intermixed with a spongy fibrous texture. This appearance of the spleen is hardly ever to be observed at a very early period of life, but is very common in middle and more advanced age I should believe that such a state of the spleen is not mark-ed by any peculiar feelings, so as to make the persons conscious of any disease taking

* Vid. Lieutaud, Tom. 1, p. 223.

place, and is probably of very little consequence in the general economy of the animal. Still, however, it is a very obvious
deviation from the healthy structure of the
spleen, and is not a state into which the
spleen naturally degenerates in the gradual
decay of the body.

The Spleen very hard.

The spleen is sometimes much harder
than natural, and at the same time is generally a good deal enlarged. When cut
into, the natural structure seems to be preserved, except that it is much more compact, the parts being much more closely
applied together.

This state of the spleen is generally considered as schirrous; and it very much resembles the hardened state of the liver, before the more common tubercles are formed
in it. I do not recollect, however, to have seen
in this state of the spleen, either schirrous
tubercles formed, or any derangement of

structure similar to schirrus in other parts of the body: it may therefore be a question, whether this is to be considered as the kind of derangement which a schirrous affection is capable of producing in this viscus, or whether it is to be considered as a disease really different. In this state of the spleen, water is sometimes accumulated in the cavity of the abdomen.

Tubercles in the Spleen.

The spleen I have seen, once or twice, studded in its substance with small tubercles, exactly similar to the scrofulous tubercles of the lungs. These were placed at pretty regular distances from each other, not running into masses; and I do not recollect to have seen any of them in a state of suppuration.

Coats of the Spleen cartilaginous.

The coats of the spleen are sometimes converted into cartilage; and this disease may be considered in a great measure as peculiar to the spleen. It is, at least, much more common in this viscus than in any other.

The cartilage is generally to be found on the convex surface of the spleen, and extends over more or less of it, in different cases. It is likewise much thicker in one case than another; in some being not thicker than a shilling, and in others being four times as thick. It is generally formed in a smooth layer, but occasionally it is somewhat irregular. It is probable, that ossifications* are sometimes to be found in this cartilage, but in the cases which have come under my own examination, bony matter was not to be observed. The cartilage into which the coats of the spleen are changed, does not resemble the cartilage at the extremities of the bones, but much more that of the nose and ears, al-

* Morgagni has seen ossification of a part of the capsule of the spleen. Vid Epist X. Art. 19 Epist. XIV. Art 23.

though it is generally of a whiter colour. This diseased process, it is natural to think, is slow in its progress, can hardly produce any impediment to the functions of the spleen, and is probably not marked by any peculiar feelings to the patient.

Spleen very large.

The spleen is sometimes found to be three or four times larger than its natural size, but with a structure perfectly healthy; and this more commonly happens to the spleen than to any other viscus. Although it may be looked upon as a monstrous growth of the spleen, rather than a disease, yet it may produce inconvenience by its pressure, and by altering in some degree the situation of the neighbouring viscera.

Hydatids are occasionally formed in the spleen,* which are of the same kind with those of the liver, but they are much more

* Vid Morgagni, Epist. XXXVIII. Art. 34.

common in the latter viscus, than in the former.

Stony concretions * have been seen occasionally in the spleen; but such cases are very rare, and have not fallen under my own observation.

The spleen has been said to be occasionally wanting, as a defect in the natural formation; but this too is very uncommon.†

* Vid. Lieutaud, Tom 1, p 231.

† Vid. Lieutaud, Tom 1, p 234

CHAP. XII.

Diseased Appearances of the Pancreas.

THE pancreas is subject to very few diseases. It seldom happens, upon examining dead bodies, that it exhibits any other than the healthy structure.

Pancreas hard.

It is not very uncommon to find the pancreas much harder than in its natural state, but without any appearance to the eye of the structure being altered. This I believe to be the beginning of a process, by which the pancreas becomes truly schirrous It very seldom in this state shews, in any part, the real schirrous structure.

I have seen this, however, to be the case, which renders it very probable, that the one is the beginning of a change into the other. When the pancreas in any part assumes the schirrous structure, that part loses entirely its natural appearance, and is converted into a hard, uniform, white mass, somewhat intersected by membrane, like schirrus in other parts of the body.

Calculi of the Pancreas.

Calculi are occasionally formed in the ducts of the pancreas. Of this I have only known one instance. The calculi were about the size of the kernel of a hazel nut, with a very irregular surface, and of a white colour. When one of the stones was put into the marine acid, it dissolved very quickly, with the extrication of a large quantity of air. The stones, therefore, in this case differed very much from the nature of urinary calculi It is probable, that calculi formed in the pancreas may differ somewhat from each other, as we find to happen in other calculi which are formed in the body; but as this is a very rare disease in the pancreas, it must be a long time before this point can be fully ascertained.

Abscesses have also been occasionally found in the pancreas, but very seldom.*

Worms have been said to have been found in its excretory duct.†

The pancreas has been said to be entirely wanting, as a defect in the original formation ‡

---

* Vid. Lieutaud, Tom. 1, p. 244.
† Vid. Lieutaud, Tom. 1, p. 248.
‡ Vid. Lieutaud, Tom. 1, p. 247.

CHAP. XIII.

*Diseased Appearances of the Kidneys, and
the Renal Capsules.*

I do not recollect to have seen the proper capsule of the kidney inflamed, and I should be inclined to consider it as a rare morbid appearance. The reason, probably, why it seldom occurs, is that the peritonæum reflected over the surface of the kidney has a very loose connection with it, there being interposed between them a considerable quantity of cellular membrane and fat. It seems very likely that the principal reason why the capsules of some other glands in the abdomen are so frequently inflamed, is their close connection with the peritonæum; and this membrane, from circumstances which perhaps it is difficult to ascertain, is very liable to inflammation.

When the capsule of the kidneys is inflamed, the same appearances of inflammation
will probably take place which have been
so often noted.

Abscesses of the Kidneys.

The substance of the kidneys is not often
inflamed without advancing to suppuration,
and perhaps there is no considerable gland
in the body so liable to form abscesses as
the kidneys. In some cases which I have
seen, the abscesses have appeared to be of
a common nature, but in the greater number of cases they have been scrofulous.

When a kidney is attacked with scrofula,
and the disease has advanced to suppuration,
it exhibits different appearances, according
to the degree of the advancement. Sometimes there are only one or two circumscribed abscesses containing a curdly pus,
without any thing being particularly observable in the inner surface of the abscesses.
Very frequently, however, the inner sur-

face of the abscesses is lined with a pulpy granulated matter. These abscesses generally first destroy the mamillary portion of the kidney; and when they advance very far, they destroy almost the whole structure of the kidney, converting it into capsules which surround a number of imperfect cavities that are lined with this pulpy substance.

The capsule into which a kidney is changed by the progress of this disease, is on some occasions thicker than on others, is frequently of considerable hardness, and seems sometimes to be laminated. At the time when a kidney is so affected, it is not uncommon for the pelvis and ureter to partake of the disease, and a calculus is often found either in the abscess, or in the pelvis of the ureter.*

* In such cases, it is very probable that the calculus is the immediate cau e of the other disease, the constitution being at the same time dis osed to t By the irritation of the calculus, inflammation and suppuration are produced in the kidney, and these partake of the nature of the constitution.

Kidney schirrous.

The kidney I have once seen converted into a firm, brown, uniform substance, somewhat intersected by membrane, in which the natural structure of this gland was entirely lost. The kidney was at the same time very much enlarged in size. This alteration of structure I should call schirrus, because it exactly resembles schirrus in other parts of the body, especially in the testicle. What effect it had upon the secretion of the urine, I have had no opportunity of being informed. This disease I am persuaded is very rare in the kidneys.

Kidneys very soft.

I have also seen the substance of the kidney converted into a soft loose mass, resembling almost exactly the appearance of common sponge. On the surface there were many round interstitial cavities scattered at irregular distances; and when the substance of the kidney was cut into, it exhibited the same spongy structure. The blood vessels of the kidney were seen ramifying very distinctly through the spongy mass. There was no appearance of pus in the kidney, nor was there the most distant resemblance between this process, and the effects produced by suppuration. It was a process of a peculiar kind, by which a considerable portion of the kidney was removed by the action, probably of absorbent vessels, and it seemed to act much more on the cortical than the tubular part of it. I am not at all exaggerating the effect of this diseased process when I say, that the kidney was rendered fully as soft as a common sponge. When shaken in water, the parts all separated from each other, somewhat like the unravelling of the shaggy vessels of the placenta Such an appearance of kidney has fallen under my observation two or three times, but I have only had once an opportunity of knowing any thing of the

symptoms which it produced during life.
I was once sent for to a woman about two
days before she died, who, besides other
ailments, complained very much of a severe
pain in the region of the kidneys, and the
urine which she passed had a very large
proportion of a sediment somewhat resembling cream How long she had complained
of these symptoms I do not now recollect,
but the time was considerable. This very
imperfect account is only thrown out to be
some guide to future inquiry, that this diseased process may be more particularly ascertained. One thing surprised me at the
time, and perhaps without reason, viz. that
this process had been attended with severe
pain. We are naturally led to expect in
processes which go on slowly, and as it
were imperceptibly, that the pain should
be inconsiderable.

Hydatids of the Kidneys.

The formation of hydatids is not an uncommon disease in the kidneys   There are
sometimes one or two considerable hydatids on the surface of a kidney, lying between its substance and capsule ; and at
other times, the natural structure of a kidney
is almost entirely lost, and is changed into
a mass of small hydatids.   When this is the
case, the mass is commonly much larger
than the natural size of a healthy kidney.
These hydatids do not appear to be of the
same nature with the hydatids of the liver
they are not inclosed in firm cysts, like
those of the liver : their coats are also
thinner, and less pulpy, and not uncommonly they are almost as thin as any membrane of the body   I do not recollect likewise to have seen any instance of small
hydatids attached to the coats of larger
hydatids in the kidney, as may be frequently observed in the liver   It is therefore

probable, that the hydatids of the kidney depend on a diseased alteration of the structure of this organ, and are not distinct organized simple animals.

Calculi of the Kidneys.

The formation of calculi is not peculiar to the kidneys, but it is a more frequent disease in them than in any other part of the body. Small granules of stone are sometimes found in the tubular portion of the kidneys, which may either be attended with inflammation, or be without it. Most commonly, however, there is found a calculus of considerable size lodged either in some part of the substance of the kidney, or in the pelvis of the ureter.

The last situation is by much the most frequent. When a stone in this situation is so large as not to be capable of passing through the ureter, it is afterwards gradually increased in size, from the contact of the urine. In its growth, it necessarily follows the branches of the pelvis, which are called infundibula, and is therefore of an arborescent form. Such calculi vary in their colour and surface; they are sometimes of a light brown, sometimes of a dark brown, and sometimes of a white colour. They are also sometimes smooth, and at other times a little roughened on their surface. Of the nature of urinary calculi we shall speak afterwards, when we come to take notice of the diseased appearances of the bladder. When a stone in the pelvis of the ureter has increased to a very considerable size, it prevents the urine almost altogether from passing into the ureter. The urine is therefore accumulated in the pelvis above the stone, and hence enlarges it very much in size, as well as the cavity of the kidney. From the pressure too of the urine behind the stone, the pelvis of the ureter, besides being enlarged, is thrust out from the substance of the kidney. If the interruption to the passage of the urine from the kidney arises from some obstruction in the lower extremity of the ureter, or at the neck of the bladder, or in any part of the urethra, not only the pelvis of the ureter is then enlarged, but the ureter itself. I have seen the ureters of both kidneys enlarged from this cause to twice or thrice their natural size.

Whatever be the nature of the obstruction, if the pelvis of the ureter be very much enlarged from the accumulation of the urine, the cavity of the kidney is at the same time enlarged. As this process advances, the substance of the kidney becomes more and more compressed, and its cavity becomes enlarged in proportion. The substance of the kidney is, at length, in a great measure lost, and is converted into a capsule, containing a great many cells, which communicate with each other. The capsule is sometimes very thin, and the whole mass is a great deal larger than the natural size of a healthy kidney. It is worthy of remark, that the urine is secreted even when the natural structure of the kidney is almost entirely lost. This is both seen in

the derangement of the kidneys now under
consideration, and when they are converted into a mass of hydatids. It would appear from this fact, that either a very small
portion of the natural structure of the kidneys is capable of secreting very nearly the
ordinary quantity of the urine; or that the
urine can be secreted by a structure that
is different from the ordinary structure of
the kidneys. Without pretending to determine this question, we shall take the liber-
ty of observing, that as the urine is a fluid
which is excrementitious, and requires only
to be separated from the blood, without
undergoing further changes like many secreted fluids, it is probable that it can be
separated by a more simple apparatus, and
under more varied circumstances, than
where the secretion from its nature must
be more complicated.

The kidneys have been said to be converted into an earthy substance.* A kid-

* Vid. Lieutaud, Tom. 1, p. 282.

ney has also been known to become ossified * Those appearances have never come under my own observation, and I am persuaded are extremely rare.

The kidneys are subject to a good deal of variety in their natural circumstances, from original formation. The two kidneys are sometimes found to be joined together: they are sometimes situated before the lumbar vertebræ, and sometimes on the sides of the pelvis They are occasionally very small in their size, and a kidney on one side is sometimes wanting ; when this is the case, the other kidney is larger than the ordinary size.

It would be very difficult to assign a satisfactory reason why there should be such variety in the kidneys, but we can see that there is no disadvantage to the animal functions produced by this variety.

The kidneys are not large in their size, and therefore may be changed in their si-

tuation without any sensible inconvenience.
As their function is independent of relative
situation, it must be precisely the same
wherever the kidneys are placed.

When the kidneys are small, the secretion
of the urine may be very nearly in the common quantity, from a greater activity in
carrying on their function ; or such persons
may be disposed to sweat more than usual,
to counterbalance the deficiency of the
urine. We know very well that the secre-
tions of the sweat and the urine are vica-
rious. When a kidney is wanting, the other,
being of a large size, is probably capable of
doing the office of two kidneys.

Diseased Appearances of the Renal Capsules.

The renal capsules are scarcely ever
found diseased. Instead of the dark coloured substance in the centre, I have sometimes seen a blackish fluid, and this is probably what is meant by authors when they
say that they have found in the cavity of a

renal capsule a fluid like ink. In such cases we may either suppose the dark coloured substance to be converted into the blackish fluid; or we may suppose that the former is removed by absorption, and the latter is deposited.

The renal capsules have been observed to contain pus.*

Little granules of stone have been found in the substance of the renal capsules †

Both of these appearances are very rare, and have not fallen under my own obser-vation.

* Vid. Lieutaud, Tom. 1, p. 285. ¦
† Vid Lieutaud, Tom. 1, p. 286,

CHAP. XIV.

Diseased Appearances of the Bladder.

Inflammation of the Peritonæal Covering.

THE bladder is covered on the outside partially by the peritonæum, which is very liable to be inflamed. That portion of it which
belongs to the bladder, is not very often inflamed by itself, but it partakes of the inflammation which extends over the membrane generally. The appearances accompanying its inflammation have been sufficiently often described. When the inflammation subsides, adhesions are frequently
left behind, connecting the bladder more or
less to the neighbouring parts ; in a female,
to the uterus, and in a male, to the rectum.

Inflammation of the inner Membrane.

The inner membrane too is sometimes inflamed. When this happens, the inflammation is either extended over the whole cavity, or is confined to a particular portion of it. The portion which is most frequently inflamed is near the neck of the bladder. This may arise from two causes; the one is, that in this situation, or near it, some obstruction is frequently found to the passage of the urine, which may produce irritation, and bring on more or less of inflammation; the other is, that inflammations of the urethra occasionally extend some way within the cavity of the bladder, and even sometimes over the whole of it. It is well known that the inner membrane of the bladder hardly shews vessels which carry red blood in its natural state, but when it is inflamed it is crowded with a prodigious number of extremely fine blood vessels, and accompanied sometimes with small spots of extra-

O

vasated blood. When the inflammation is in a high degree, the muscular coat of the bladder may be affected ; but as this is only loosely attached to the inner membrane, the inflammation will not very readily pass from the one to the other.

Ulcers.

Inflammation of the inner membrane of the bladder advances sometimes to the formation of pus, and abscesses and ulcers are occasionally produced These, when the inflammation has been of the common sort, exhibit the ordinary appearances which have been often mentioned. They sometimes advance so far as to destroy a portion of the bladder entirely, and to form communications between it and the neighbouring parts, as with the general cavity of the abdomen, with the rectum in the male, and the vagina in the female When the communication is formed with the general cavity of the abdomen, the urine escapes into

it, producing there general peritonæal inflammation, of which I recollect a very
striking example. When the communication is formed with the vagina or the rectum, the urine will escape by these passages,
producing in them more or less of irritation
and inflammation.

When abscesses take place in the bladder,
they are produced more frequently from
local violence, than from a previous spontaneous inflammation. One of the most
common causes of violence is the incision of
the bladder in the operation of lithotomy.
When the part has been very much irritated in the operation, or the constitution is
such that it is excited into violent action
from the common degree of irritation, an
ulcer is formed at the lips of the wound, and
spreads more or less into the cavity of the
bladder.

It sometimes happens, although I believe
very rarely, that the whole of the inner
membrane of the bladder is destroyed by
ulceration, and its muscular fibres appear

as bare as if they had been nicely dissected.
In the case where I recollect this process to have taken place most completely,
the bladder was almost filled with a scrofulous pus. This had exactly the same appearance as when a scrofulous absorbent
gland suppurates, viz. there was a curdly
white matter mixed with pus.

Schirrus and Cancer.

I do not think that schirrus or cancer often attack the bladder by itself, but it
sometimes partakes of this disease from its
contiguity to parts which are very liable to
it The disease on some occasions spreads to
the bladder from the rectum, and on others
from the uterus: under such circumstances
the bladder becomes very thick and hard,
and exhibits the ordinary cancerous structure. Communications too are generally
formed either with the rectum, the uterus,
or the vagina.

Fungous Excrescences.

Sometimes fungous excrescences arise from the inner surface of the bladder, either in one mass, or in separate portions. When examined, they are found to consist of a loose fibrous structure. When they are situated a little behind the neck of the bladder, which is not uncommonly the case, they must produce a considerable obstruction to the passage of the urine. A stronger action will, therefore, be required in the bladder to expel the urine, and its muscular coat will be consequently thickened: accordingly it is frequently found thickened ; and it is not improbable that even where the situation of the fungus may not obstruct the passage of the urine into the urethra, its presence may still irritate the bladder so as to excite it to more frequent and stronger actions than in a natural state, and the muscular coat become thereby thickened.

Elongations of the inner Membrane.

I have also known the inner membrane of the bladder elongated in some parts, so as to form irregular processes. These when cut into, were found to consist of a considerable quantity of cellular membrane, intermixed with a little fat The process producing such an appearance was probably a slow one, and was probably also attended with no pain. If these elongations were to be situated at a distance from the neck of the bladder, one can hardly perceive how they could produce any inconvenience, but if situated near the neck of the bladder, they might occasion extreme difficulty in making water, and even lay the foundation of a fatal disease.

Muscular Coat thickened.

One of the most ordinary changes in the bladder, from its natural structure, is the great thickening of its muscular coat. In a natural state, the muscular coat of the bladder (when it is moderately distended) consists of thin layers of muscular fibres, running in different directions. These are probably altogether, not more than the eighth of an inch in thickness. The muscular coat of the bladder, however, is occasionally found at least half an inch thick. This arises from an additional quantity of muscle being formed in consequence of extraordinary efforts being necessary in the bladder. These efforts take place when there is any considerable difficulty in making water, as happens when the prostate gland is a good deal enlarged, when there is a stone in the bladder, or when there are strictures of the urethra. It is usual, therefore, to find this thickening of the muscular coat of the bladder when there is any of these diseases. When the bladder is thickened, the fasciculi of which its muscular coat is composed become much larger, but never, or at least very seldom, acquire the full red colour which muscles have in other parts of the body.

This is a deviation from the general plan of nature with regard to the increase of muscles from exercise. When muscles are enlarged in size from exercise, they also become of a deep red colour. There is no other instance too in the body, as far as I recollect, of a muscle being so much enlarged beyond its natural size in consequence of increased exertion, as the muscular coat of the bladder. Between the fasciculi of the muscular fibres, little pouches are formed by the inner membrane This arises from the pressure of the urine against the inner membrane of the bladder which is impelled by the strong powers of the muscular coat. These pouches are often large enough to admit the end of the finger, and contain occasionally small calculi. The bladder in this state admits of very little distension, so that it is capable of containing little water; hence the inclination to make water is frequent, and frequent efforts of the muscular coat are required, which increase more and more its thickness. It is much more com-

mon to find this appearance of the bladder
in the male than in the female, because in
the latter there are fewer causes to produce
it There is in that sex a want of the prostate gland altogether, and the urethra being
short and wide, obstructions seldom take
place in it. When the muscular coat of the
bladder is thickened, I believe that it has
been sometimes mistaken for schirrus.

Calculi.

Calculi are not uncommonly found in the
bladder, and are confined in their formation to no particular period of life. They
are formed in very young children, and also in persons of middle and advanced age.
This disease is not so frequently met with
in the female as in the male, which may
depend on two causes ; the one is, that
there is not so strong a tendency to their
formation in that sex ; and the other cause
is, that stones escape through the urethra
in women, which would be detained in the

bladder of men, and lay the foundation there of larger calculi.

The stones which are found in the bladder, are either originally formed in the kidneys, and pass through the ureters into the bladder, or they are first formed in the bladder itself. When the last circumstance takes place, the earthy matter is sometimes first deposited round some extraneous body, which becomes the nucleus of the calculus, although most frequently no nucleus whatever is to be observed. The nuclei which I have seen have been small portions of lead (probably broken off from a leaden bougie) small nails, and little masses of hair In short, any extraneous body which may happen to be introduced into the bladder, may become a nucleus It is natural to think that such nuclei are more common in the calculi found in the bladder of women, than of men ; their urethra is wider and shorter, so that an extraneous body can be much more easily introduced into the bladder , and women too, from the particular frame of their minds, are more apt to make experiments of this sort than men.

The calculi of the bladder either lie loose in it, or are confined to some fixed situation, from particular circumstances. When they are of a small size, they are sometimes lodged in pouches, or sacculi, formed by the protrusion of the inner membrane of the bladder between the fasciculi of its muscular fibres. A calculus also is occasionally attached to an excrescence of the bladder, so as to be kept in a fixed situation.

There is frequently one calculus only in the bladder at a time, and then it is usually of an oval form; but there are often more, and the calculi by rubbing upon each other acquire flat sides and angles. Calculi have sometimes a smooth uniform surface, but most frequently the surface is granulated. These granules are commonly placed very near each other over the whole surface of the calculus, giving it a certain degree of roughness. I have also seen them gathered into clusters on particular parts of the surface of a calculus. These granules are also sometimes of a smaller, at other times of a larger size, and in different calculi are more or less elevated. Some calculi have an irregular porous structure upon the surface, instead of being granulated.

Caluli when divided by the saw, or broken, exhibit most commonly a laminated structure. These laminæ are disposed in concentric curves, and are applied together with more or less compactness. They also differ in their thickness in different calculi: the laminated structure sometimes pervades uniformly the whole mass of the calculus; at other times different portions of it are interrupted by a coarse porous texture. In some calculi no laminated structure whatever is observable, but it is entirely porous.

The colour of calculi varies considerably. They are most frequently of a brown colour, which is sometimes of a lighter, and

at other times of a darker shade. They
are also sometimes of a white, and often
of a yellowish colour. It is remarkable,
that different portions of the same calculus
are frequently of a different colour. Some
laminæ, for instance, are perfectly white,
while the other laminæ are brown. In this
sort of mixture, I have most commonly
found the white laminæ on the outside, and
the brown laminæ in the middle; and I do
not recollect seeing one instance of laminæ
of different colours, disposed in alternate
strata.

The specific gravity of urinary calculi
differs very considerably, as they differ a
good deal in their compactness; but they
are generally a little more than twice the
specific gravity of water.

The chemical properties of different urinary calculi, I am apt to believe, differ more
from each other than has generally been
imagined. Any trials which I have made
have led me to this opinion; but I am so
little accustomed to chemical experiments

that I do not rest upon it with much confidence.

The celebrated Scheele made a number of experiments to ascertain the nature of urinary calculi, of which the following are the chief.

1. Diluted vitriolic acid does not act on urinary calculi at all, but the concentrated dissolves them in heat.

2. Marine acid, whether diluted or concentrated, does not act on urinary calculi, not even when boiled with them.*

3. Nitrous acid diluted, or aqua fortis, act a little on urinary calculi in the cold, but on the application of heat act with effervescence and with vapours.

4 This solution tinges the skin with deep red spots within half an hour after being applied, is not precipitated by alkalis, but on the application of lime-water yields a white precipitate.

* I have met with an urinary calculus capable of being dissolved in marine acid, even in the common temperature of the atmosphere.

5. Ponderous earth dissolved in marine acid, does not occasion any precipitate from this solution.

6. Acid of sugar, or salt of sorrel, does not produce any precipitate from this solution.

7. A calculus when pounded and boiled in a solution of alkali of tartar, remains unchanged ; but perfectly pure, or caustic alkali, such as does not shew the least mark of the aerial acid, dissolves the calculus even in the cold.

8 Lime-water dissolves the urinary calculus, by digestion, in the proportion of four ounces of lime-water to twelve grains of the calculus.

9. Pure water dissolves an urinary calculus, in the proportion of five ounces of the water to eight grains of the calculus ; and this solution changes the tincture of lacmus to a red colour.

10 On distilling, in a small glass retort, one drachm of calculus in the open fire, there was obtained a volatile alkaline liquor

like that of hartshorn, but no oil. In the neck of the retort there was a brown subli-mate. Upon heating the retort thoroughly red hot, and then leaving it to cool, there was obtained a black coal, weighing twelve grains, which when put upon red hot iron in the open air, retained its black colour The sublimate, which seemed to have been somewhat fused, weighed twenty-eight grains; and upon being purified by a new sublimation, it grew white. It had no smell, but a somewhat sourish taste, and was easily soluble in boiling water. it also dissolved in spirit of wine, but a larger quantity than of water was requisite for this purpose Lime-water was not precipitated The sublimate seemed to agree in some respects with the sal succini.

From these and some other experiments Scheele concludes, that urinary calculi are neither gypseous nor calcareous, but consist of an oily, dry, volatile acid concrete, mix-ed with some gelatinous matter.

Bergman, by burning the charcoal of

urinary calculi to a white cinder, obtained some calcareous earth, and calculates that the proportion of it in these stones is about $\frac{1}{200}$ part.

Although the world is much obliged to these two celebrated chemists, Scheele and Bergman, for their labours upon this as well as many other subjects, yet I am inclined to think that a sufficient number of urinary calculi has not yet been examined, to ascertain all the variety of their constituent parts.

Although the matter of calculus in the bladder is generally formed into one or more circumscribed masses, yet I have seen the whole bladder filled with a substance like mortar. This could not be removed entirely from it; but a great many small irregular portions still adhered to the sides of its cavity I believe this matter to have been of the same nature with a common calculus, because it exhibited the same affinities with the common acids.

In opening dead bodies, the bladder is

P

occasionally found to be very much distended, and to occupy the lower part of the cavity of the abdomen. This might arise from some accidental circumstance of the water being accumulated, while the muscular coat of the bladder still possessed its proper powers; or the muscular coat of the bladder may have been paralytic, and therefore not capable of expelling the water. I do not think it is possible to discriminate between these two different situations by any examination after death, but they can always be ascertained by inquiry into the history of the case

The bladder is also found contracted to such a degree as hardly to have any cavity. This is generally not to be considered as a disease, but simply as having arisen from a very strong action of the muscular coat of the bladder previously to death.

The anterior part of the bladder is occasionally found wanting, and instead of it there is a very soft vascular flesh, situated externally at the lower part of the abdomen.

This soft vascular flesh is usually formed
into irregular projecting masses, and in the
living body is covered with a thick ropy
mucus. The two ureters open somewhere
upon this vascular flesh, distilling gradually
the urine as it is secreted upon its surface,
which the mucus is intended to protect
against the stimulus of that fluid. When
there is such a formation of the bladder, I
believe that there is always found a deficiency of the bone at the symphysis pubis,
and also a monstrous formation of some of
the organs of generation. This species of
monstrosity I have described at large in the
Medical and Chirurgical Transactions.*

Another kind of monstrous formation in
the bladder occasionally happens, viz. that
at its depending part there is a communication between it and the rectum, the latter
being continued into the former. Of this I
have seen one instance, and it has been already taken notice of, when treating of the

* See Medical and Chirurgical Transactions, p 189.

diseased and preternatural appearances of the intestines.

A portion of the bladder at its fundus, has been known to be lodged in a hernial sack, both at the abdominal ring and under Paupart's ligament; but this is very rare, and has not fallen under my own observation.*

* See Pott on Ruptures, p. 226.

CHAP. XV.

Diseased Appearances of the Vesiculæ Seminales.

THE diseased appearances of the vesiculæ seminales are not very commonly known, because from their situation these bodies cannot be seen without a good deal of dissection ; whereas many of the viscera come immediately into view when the cavity is simply laid open in which they are lodged: diseased appearances, however, have been occasionally observed in them.

It has never occurred to me, to observe the vesiculæ seminales inflamed by themselves, although they are, no doubt, liable to this disease like every other part of the body. I have seen them, however, involved in the natural consequences of inflammation with the surrounding parts. Thus I have seen the posterior surface of the bladder, the vesiculæ seminales, and a portion of the rectum adhering with unusual firmness together, in the same manner as other parts of the body frequently do after inflammation.

The vesiculæ seminales are also affected with scrofula. Upon one occasion I recollect to have seen one of the vesiculæ seminales filled with true scrofulous matter, the distinguishing characteristic of which has been often mentioned.

The ducts of the vesiculæ seminales open naturally by two distinct orifices into the cavity of the prostate gland, but they are occasionally wanting, and the vesiculæ seminales terminate in a cul-de-sac. The vasa deferentia are at the same time without their natural termination, for they end in the cul-de-sac of the vesiculæ seminales This is a species of monstrosity which is very rare, but it is of great consequence, because it prevents the semen from passing into the urethra, and frustrates one of the most important functions in the animal economy.

The vesiculæ seminales differ a good deal in their size in different adult bodies, and indeed it is very common for the one to be considerably smaller than the other; but I have oftener than once seen both of them so small that they must have been very little able to fulfil the intentions for which they were formed.

One of the vesiculæ seminales is occasionally wanting altogether. Under such circumstances I should believe that the extremity of the vas deferens upon that side is most frequently enlarged and tortuous, becoming a sort of substitute for it. This was at least the case in the instance which I have seen of this mode of formation. The extremity of the vas deferens has at all times a structure similar to that of the vesiculæ seminales, and renders therefore this conjecture very probable.

The vesiculæ seminales have also been observed to be schirrous; but this is not at all common.*

* See Morgagni, Epist. XLVI. Art. 5.

CHAP. XVI.

Diseased Appearances of the Prostate Gland.

Abscess in the Prostate Gland.

THE prostate gland is not often found in a state of common inflammation. I have seen, however, an abscess in it, without any uncommon thickening and enlargement of the gland, and where the pus appeared to be of the common sort. This must be considered as being a common abscess, and must have been preceded by the ordinary sort of inflammation.

Scrofula of the Prostate Gland.

The prostate gland is sometimes scrofulous I have seen, in cutting into it, precisely the same white curdly matter, which takes place in a scrofulous absorbent gland. In squeezing it also, I have forced out from its ducts a scrofulous pus.

Schirrus of the Prostate Gland.

The most common disease of the prostate gland is a schirrous enlargement of it. The prostate gland, it is well known, is naturally about the size of a large chesnut, but when it is attacked by schirrus, it is often enlarged to the size of the fist. In this enlarged state, the external appearance of its structure is not different from what is natural, but when cut into, it exhibits a very firm, whitish, or brown substance, with membranous septa running through it in various directions, which are often very strongly marked This is the appearance of schirrus in other parts of the body. When the prostate gland is a good deal enlarged, its cavity becomes deeper from the growth of its sides, and the posterior extremity forms a considerable projection into the cavity of the bladder, which interrupts the passage of the urine into the urethra. According to the degree of this projection, the urine is passed with greater or less difficulty, as well as an instrument for drawing it off. When the projection is very great, it has sometimes been found impossible to pass an instrument over the projection, and an artificial passage has occasionally been made through it accidentally, by which the urine has been evacuated. Under such circumstances the gland has been known not to be irritated by the violence used in making this new passage, and life has been prolonged for a greater length of time than it would have been otherwise. Still, however, the instrument ought to be made to pass over the projection, if possible; and we should never run the risk, by injuring the gland, of bringing on immediate fatal consequences.

Sometimes in the progress of the enlargement the prostate gland grows irregularly, and a winding passage is formed through it,

by an alteration in the shape of its cavity.
This increases the difficulty to the patient
of making water, and to the surgeon of in-
troducing an instrument When the prostate gland is enlarged, its internal surface
is sometimes ulcerated, but commonly it is
not. Fistulous communications are sometimes formed between an enlarged prostate gland and the rectum. It is obvious
too, from what has been mentioned, that in
an enlarged state of the prostate gland, the
difficulty of making water must be very
great. This difficulty excites extraordinary
and very frequent efforts in the bladder to
overcome it Its muscular coat becomes
consequently much stronger and thickened
A prostate gland, therefore, is never found
enlarged to any considerable degree, without the bladder having undergone this
change in its muscular coat. This disease
is hardly ever to be found in a young person, but is not at all uncommon at an advanced period of life

Calculi in the Ducts of the Prostate Gland.

There is another disease of the prostate gland, which occasionally takes place, although it is by no means so frequent as the former, viz. a formation of small calculi, which are lodged in its ducts. They are usually of the size of a small pea, and those which I have seen have been of a brown or black colour. What is their exact nature I cannot positively ascertain, because to do this requires a much nicer management of chemical experiments than I pretend to possess, but from some very imperfect trials which I have made, they seemed to differ in their properties from urinary calculi.* What I say, however, relates only to the brown calculi; with regard to the other, I have had no opportunity of examining them.

* They were almost entirely dissolved in the vitriolic acid, but were only separated into a fine powder by the nitrous.

Ducts of the Prostate Gland enlarged.

The prostate gland is sometimes seen with its cavity very much widened, and its ducts enlarged. In the natural state of the gland, the orifices of its ducts can hardly be seen, but they sometimes are so much enlarged as to be capable of admitting a crow quill. When the ducts are so enlarged, there is always a great obstruction to the passage of the urine through the urethra, arising most commonly from stricture there. The urine, either passing in very small quantity, or being entirely obstructed, is accumulated in the cavity of the prostate gland and the bladder. The effect of this accumulation is, that the cavity of the prostate gland is widened, and the ducts very much enlarged. The bladder too, from making extraordinary efforts to overcome the obstruction, has its muscular coat gradually thickened, and often to a very considerable degree. Attending, therefore, this

state of the prostate gland there is a thickened bladder, and an obstructed urethra.

The *Prostate Gland preternaturally small.*

I have also seen the prostate gland of an
extremely small size, so that one could
hardly suppose it from this circumstance to
be fit for its office. It was attended with a
monstrous formation of the urinary bladder
and some of the organs of generation, and
has been particularly described by me in the
Medical and Chirurgical Transactions. *

* See p. 194.

CHAP. XVII.

Diseased Appearances of the Urethra.

Abscesses.

ABSCESSES are occasionally formed in the membranous part of the urethra. These may arise from an inflammation, produced by some latent cause, as abscesses are formed in any other part of the body; but they happen most frequently from an obstruction to the passage of urine through the urethra. This obstruction is produced generally by a stricture in some part of this canal, but most frequently it is a little anterior to the membranous portion of it. The urine being forced by the efforts of the bladder behind the stricture, irritates that part, producing inflammation and suppuration, the abscess breaks externally, and the urine is evacuated by this opening. While it remains in the state of an abscess, it is not at all different from any common abscess which may communicate with the bladder.

Fistulæ.

While the obstruction in the urethra continues, the opening made by the breaking of the abscess is not allowed to close, but a fistulous orifice is gradually formed. This is surrounded with parts somewhat thickened and hard, as fistulæ are generally. The most common situation for these fistulous openings is behind the scrotum, near the membranous part of the urethra, because the most common situation of the stricture is a little anterior to this part of the urethra. Not uncommonly there are more than one of these openings leading to short canals which run in different directions.

The membranous part of the urethra I have also seen formed into a bag large enough to contain a hen's egg, and consisting of a pretty firm substance., This bag was occasioned by a large stone which had lodged there.

I do not recollect to have seen Cowper's glands diseased, which are situated near this part of the urethra. They must be liable to changes from disease, like other parts of the body; but they are small and difficult of access, so that they have very seldom become an object of examination

Morgagni mentions one of them being converted into a ligamentous substance;* and one of the excretory ducts in another instance being obliterated.†

The inner membrane of the urethra is very liable to be inflamed, particularly at its anterior extremity, and the inflammation occasionally spreads over the whole extent of the canal. This exhibits no appearance different from the inflammation of membranes lining secretory canals which open externally. The inner membrane of

* See Morgagni, Epist XLIV. Art 3.
† See Morgagni, Epist XLIV. Art. 12.

the urethra is much more crowded with small blood vessels than in a natural state, and there is an increased secretion of the glands which open upon it. The inflammation is often not confined to the inner membrane of the urethra, but spreads into the substance of the corpus spongiosum, affecting both its cellular structure and its glands. Under these circumstances, the corpus spongiosum is enlarged and harder from the extravasation of the coagulable lymph into its cells, and is more vascular than in a natural state. The glands being increased in size from the inflammation, become sensible to the touch, like very small rounded tubercles.

Ulcers are also seen occasionally in laying open the urethra, but these are not frequent

Stricture.

The most ordinary diseased appearance of the urethra is stricture This consists in a part of the canal being narrowed, or perhaps altogether obliterated. It may take place in any part of the canal, but it is most frequent a little anterior to the membranous part of the urethra. This stricture consists sometimes of an approximation simply of the opposite sides of the canal, so as to form a line of obstruction, and at other times the canal is narrowed for some length. The inner membrane, at the stricture, sometimes exhibits the natural appearance of surface ; at other times the surface is abraded or ulcerated These effects are generally produced by bougies, and sometimes false passages have been made into the corpus spongiosum urethræ in consequence of employing too much violence in the use of this instrument. There is very commonly more than one stricture in the same urethra It sometimes happens too, that the stricture is more on one side of the canal than the other, so that the passage there is crooked.

Caruncle.

A small fleshy excrescence sometimes grows in the urethra. This is called caruncle, and used formerly to be considered as the most common cause of obstruction in this canal, but since dissections of dead bodies have become more frequent, it has been found in reality to be very rare.

I have known one instance of a thin layer of earthy matter extending from the bladder through the whole length of the urethra.

Preternatural Orifice of the Urethra.

The urethra sometimes does not open at the projecting extremity of the glans penis, but under it, where the frenum is naturally situated; and in such cases there is no frenum. It consists of a small rounded opening, much less than when there is the natural termination in the glans. I have known an

instance in this structure of parts, of a canal being formed besides the urethra, about
two inches in length, which terminated at
one extremity in a cul-de-sac, and at the
other opened on the glans where the urethra commonly does. How far this variety
may be frequent, I cannot pretend to determine. This deviation in the structure is
not to be considered as a disease, but simply
as a mal-formation of parts, and is not attended with any material inconvenience, as
far as I know

There are some other diseased appearances of the penis, such as ulcers, phymo-
ses, paraphymosis, &c These are external,
are very well known, and do not properly
fall within my plan ; I shall therefore omit
them entirely.

CHAP. XVIII.

Diseased Appearances of the Testicles, and the Spermatic Chord.

Hydrocele.

HYDROCELE, or a collection of water in the tunica vaginalis testis, is a very common complaint, and is confined to no particular period of life. It is not unfrequent in very young children, and in them most commonly disappears without any chirurgical treatment. In persons who are grown up, the disease scarcely ever goes away spontaneously, but requires the assistance of art. The bag in which the water is accumulated is of a pyramidal shape, and approaches more or less towards the ring of the abdominal muscle, according to the degree of the accumulation. It sometimes extends almost to the ring itself. The bag is also more or less thick in different cases. it is often scarcely thicker than the tunica vaginalis in its natural state; at other times, when the accumulation is large, it is three or four times thicker, and is obviously laminated. In such cases too the testicle is a good deal compressed, and has sometimes been known to waste in consequence of this compression. The fluid which is accumulated is of a yellowish, a greenish, or brown colour, and resembles in its properties the serum of the blood. This disease, in persons who are advanced in life, is frequently combined with a schirrous state of the testicle, which will be afterwards particularly explained.

Hydatids.

Hydatids have sometimes been found in the cavity of the tunica vaginalis testis, either loose or adhering; but I have had no opportunity of examining them, and they are not at all common.*

Adhesions.

The tunica vaginalis is frequently found adhering to the surface of the testicle. The adhesion is sometimes extended over the whole surface, but frequently consists only of scattered processes of membrane. The adhesions are sometimes fine, but at other times have considerable thickness, and connect the tunica vaginalis to the body of the testicle more or less closely in different cases. They are produced by some previous inflammation, as in the cavity of the chest and belly; but it does not often occur that a tunica vaginalis is examined after death, which immediately before had been in an active state of inflammation.

* See Morgagni, Epist. IV. Art. 30.

Testicle inflamed.

The substance of the testicle itself is very frequently inflamed, but this is commonly removed by art, and therefore hardly ever becomes an object of examination after death It exhibits, however, precisely the same appearances as the inflammation of the substance of other parts, and therefore does not require to be particularly described. When the testicle is inflamed, the vas deferens sometimes partakes of the inflammation, its coats becoming considerably thickened, and in some instances the veins of the spermatic chord have been known to become varicose * After the inflammation of the testicle has subsided, it is not unusual for a hardness and fullness of the epidydimis to remain for a considerable length of time, or even through life This depends on the matter which had been extravasated

* See Mr Hunter on the Venereal Disease, p. 54

during the inflammation not being afterwards entirely absorbed.

Abscesses too are not unfrequently formed in the testicles, from the progress of common inflammation, and are attended with the same circumstances as abscesses in other parts.

Testicle scrofulous.

The testicle is sometimes completely changed from its natural structure, and converted into a mass of truly scrofulous substance. Upon such occasions it is generally enlarged in its size, and when cut into, shews a white, or yellowish white, curdly substance, which is sometimes more or less mixed with pus.

Testicle enlarged and pulpy.

The testicle is sometimes much enlarged in size, and converted into a brown, uniform, pulpy matter, in which its natural structure

is entirely lost. This sort of change has
been sometimes mistaken for schirrus, although it is very different from what is called schirrus in other parts of the body, and
what is also found in the testicle itself.

Schirrus and Cancer of the Testicle.

The testicle is often found much enlarged,
where its natural structure is lost, and
where it is changed into a hard mass of a
brownish colour, which is generally more or
less intersected by membrane. There is
sometimes mixed in this structure cartilage;
and sometimes there are cells formed in it
containing a sanious fluid. This state of
the testicle I consider as the true schirrus,
and according to the progress of the disease,
the epidydimis and the spermatic chord
are more or less, or not at all, affected. This
disease not unfrequently advances to form
a foul deep ulcer, or throws out a fungus,
and then it is called the true cancer of the
testicle.

Testicle cartilaginous.

The testicle I have seen much enlarged in size, and changed into a mass of cartilage. This does not seem different in any essential property from common cartilage, but is only a little softer. This I should consider as depending upon the same general diseased process with the schirrus just described, for sometimes both structures are blended together in the same testicle.

Testicle bony.

The testicle is sometimes converted into bone. This is not a very unfrequent disease, and is more commonly confined to some part of the testicle, than extended over the whole of it.

I have seen a testicle with a small firm cyst adhering to it, which contained a worm of that sort called vena medinensis. This is a worm of considerable length, with

a smooth surface, and an uniform appearance; at the posterior extremity it terminates in a slender hook-like process, and at
the anterior, there is a rounded opening or
mouth. It very commonly burrows under
the skin of the inhabitants of some warm
countries, particularly Guinea, and is very
troublesome *to* them This testicle had
probably belonged to a man who had visit-
ed some of those climates in which the vena medinensis is found, and who had
brought it over with him to this country.

The Epidydimis ending in a Cul-de-Sac.

The testicles have sometimes this sort of
mal-formation, that the epidydimis does not
terminate in a vas deferens, but in a cul-de-
sac. In these cases it is evident that the
semen can never be evacuated by the urethra, and the person must therefore be incapable of procreation.

Stricture of the Vas Deferens.

I have also seen a portion of the canal of the vas deferens obliterated by stricture. This had not been an original fault, but was the effect of a diseased process, and must have prevented the semen of that testicle from reaching the urethra.

Testicles very small, and wasted.

The testicles are sometimes exceedingly small in their size. I have known one case, in a person of middle age, where each of them was not larger than the extremity of the finger of an adult This, as appeared from its history, arose from a fault in the original formation, and was attended with a total want of the natural propensities. It is much more common for a testicle to waste either spontaneously, or in consequence of a former inflammation, or compression, so

as gradually to disappear entirely.* When
this takes place in one testicle only, the natural powers are preserved, but when it
takes place in both, they must be altogether lost.

Sometimes one testicle, and sometimes
both remain in the cavity of the abdomen
through life, so that a person appears to
have only one testicle, or to be without them
altogether. The testicle or testicles, I believe, in these cases are of a small size, and
Mr. Hunter suspects that they are by no
means so perfect as when they descend
into the scrotum.†

Diseased Appearances of the Spermatic Chord.

The spermatic chord is also liable to diseased alterations of structure : one of the
most common is that of its becoming schir-

* See Hunter on the Venereal Disease, p. 209

† See Mr. Hunter's Observations on certain Parts of the
Animal Economy, p 18.

rous. This I believe to be very rarely, if at all an original disease of the chord, but always, or almost always, spreads to it from the testicle. In the early state of a schirrous testicle the spermatic chord is perfectly sound, and this is the proper season for the extirpation of the testicle; but when the disease has taken place for a considerable time, and does not remain stationary, the chord becomes at length affected. Under such circumstances it is changed into a large hard mass, exhibiting the same appearance of structure with the testicle itself During the last stage the disease advances to the loins, so as to affect the absorbent glands there.

When the testicle is scrofulous, the spermatic chord sometimes partakes of the same disease, and exhibits also the same appearance of change with the testicle itself.

A disease of the spermatic chord which is not uncommon, is an enlargement of its veins. The veins of the spermatic chord are numerous, and support a very long column of blood. This last circumstance,

R

added to some impediments which occasion-
al'y take place to obstruct the return of the
blood, renders the veins frequently enlarged. This enlargement varies very much
in different cases, arising from the degree
and the continuance of the impediment.
When the enlargement of the veins is very
considerable, they also become varicose, and
the spermatic chord is changed into a bulky
mass, soft to the feeling, and capable of being readily diminished upon pressure. In
this state of the spermatic chord, the testicle is sometimes wasted.

Wa'er has sometimes been known to be
accumulated in the cells of the cellular membrane, which envelopes the vessels of the
spermatic chord. The cellular membrane of
this part of the body is in considerable quantity, and when water is accumulated in its
cells, there is a large swelling formed in
the situation of the spermatic chord, which
is readily diminished upon pressure. When
pressure is used, the swelling is diminished,
not only by a part of the water being forced

into the cells of the chord within the abdominal ring, but also by its being forced into the cellular membrane under the skin of the lower part of the belly. Many pints have been known to be accumulated in these cells. It has never occurred to myself to see this disease, and therefore I have had no opportunity of examining the nature of the fluid, but I presume it is of the same sort with what is usually found in anasarca.

A sack has also been known to be formed in the spermatic chord, consisting of a firm white membrane, and containing a fluid which most probably is of a serous nature. Both of these cases have been particularly described by Mr. Pott in his Treatise upon Hydrocele.*

* For the first case, see Pott on Hydrocele, p. 39. For the second, see Pott on Hydrocele, p. 57.

CHAP. XIX.

Diseased Appearances in the Female Organs.

Inflammation of the Uterus.

WHEN the uterus is inflamed, it takes place almost always under the same circumstances, viz very soon after parturition. The inflammation is sometimes confined to the uterus itself, or its appendages, but the peritonæum in the neighbourhood is most commonly affected, and frequently over the whole extent of the cavity of the abdomen The uterus when inflamed, exhibits the same appearances as the inflammation of the substance of other parts, and these are principally observable in its body or fundus. The inflammation is frequently found to creep along the appendages of the uterus, especially the Fallopian tubes and ovaria It often advances to suppuration, and the pus is generally found in the large veins of the womb.* When the peritonæum is also affected by inflammation, it exhibits the same appearances which we formerly described particularly, when treating of the inflammation of this membrane; but the extravasated fluid, and the coagulable lymph, are not uncommonly in very large proportion to the degree of the inflammation †

Schirrus of the Uterus.

One of the most frequent diseases of the uterus is schirrus. In this state it is increased more or less in bulk, and often to a very large size. Its substance when cut into is thick and hard, and when its structure is examined, it shews a whitish firm substance,

* See Dr. Clarke's Essays, p. 69 and 70.

† Dr Clarke, who has examined a great many women that have died after parturition with inflammation of the peritonæum, has observed this particularly. See **Dr. Clarke's** Essays, p. 136

intersected generally by strong membranous divisions. This is the common appearance of the structure of schirrus in other parts, and it differs less from the natural appearance of the structure of the uterus than that of any other part of the body. In this state of the uterus, its internal surface is commonly found ulcerated, forming cancer, and sometimes so much so as to throw out long ragged processes. The ulceration also sometimes extends to the neighbouring parts, as the vagina, the bladder, and the rectum, making communications between them, and producing dreadful havock. The uterus is occasionally almost entirely destroyed by the progress of the disease I have seen several instances where the fundus of the uterus only was remaining, and where the rest was changed into a tattered ulcerated mass.

It is worthy of remark, that schirrus or cancer attacks generally the cervix uteri before the fundus This may perhaps depend upon a general principle, which we have often mentioned : the cervix uteri is more glandular than any other part of the uterus, and schirrus or cancer appears to be peculiarly a disease of glandular parts.

Tubercles of the Uterus

Hard tubercles often grow from the uterus, which are either imbedded in its substance, or arise from its outer surface. They vary a good deal in their size, viz. from that of a hazel nut to more than the size of the fist. They are irregular in their shape, but are commonly rounded, and are in some degree tuberculated. These when cut into, shew a whitish very firm substance, intersected by membranous septa, which are commonly very thick and strong. It is extremely rare that those circumscribed masses are found ulcerated. The uterus in this state of disease is generally of the natural size.

A mass of the same kind is sometimes found in the cavity of the uterus, and often grows to a very large size   I have seen it a good deal larger than a child's head at birth This mass when cut into, exhibits precisely the same appearances which we have so lately described It is remarkable, that those masses within the cavity of the uterus commonly do not adhere in any part closely to it, but are connected with it loosely, by the intervention of the cellular membrane, so that they can be very easily peeled off, without injuring the structure of the uterus The uterus itself is more or less enlarged according to the bulk of the mass it contains, but appears to be perfectly healthy in its structure

Polypus.

Polypus forms a very common disease of the uterus, and may take place almost at any period of life ; it is more frequent, however, at the middle or advanced age, and very rarely happens in persons who are young By a polypus is meant a diseased mass, which adheres to some part of the cavity of the uterus, by a sort of neck or narrower portion It is of different kinds : the most common kind is hard, and consists evidently of a white substance, divided by very thick membranous septa. When cut into, it shews precisely the same structure with the tubercle of the uterus lately described ; so that a person looking upon a section of the one and the other, out of the body, could not at all distinguish between them. This sort of polypus varies very much in its size, some being not larger than a walnut, and others being larger than a child's head. It adheres by a narrower portion or neck, which varies a great deal in its size, and in its proportion to the body of the polypus. The largest polypus I ever saw was suspended by a neck hardly thicker than the thumb ; and I have seen a polypus, much less than the fist, adhering by a neck fully as thick as the wrist.

The place of adhesion also differs considerably It is most commonly at the fundus uteri, but it may take place in any other part ; and I have seen a small polypus adhering just on the inner part of the lip of the os uteri. When a polyus is of any considerable size, there is generally but one ; but I have occasionally seen on the inside of the uterus, two or three small polypi. Another sort of polypus takes place in the uterus, which consists of a bulky, irregular, bloody mass, with a number of tattered processes hanging from it. This when cut into exhibits two different appearances of structure : the one appearance is that of a spongy mass, consisting of laminæ, with small interstitial cavities between them ; the other is that of a very loose texture, consisting of large irregular cavities These are the different varieties in polypi, which I have observed, but perhaps there may be others, which have not come under my notice It is very obvious, that in proportion as a polypus grows, the cavity of the uterus must be enlarged, and the same change must take place in the vagina, when a polypus leaves the uterus, and passes into this canal.

The Inversion of the Uterus.

The inversion of the uterus occasionally takes place, and principally from two causes, viz. from the weight of a polypus, or from violent pulling in attempts to remove the placenta. When the inversion is incomplete, the fundus uteri forms a tumour within its cavity ; there is at the same time an appearance of fissure upon the outside of the uterus, where the fundus usually is ; and the Fallopian tubes, round ligaments, and ligaments of the ovaria, are drawn inwards at both edges of the fissure. The uterus, particularly after labour, is sometimes inverted entirely, the inner surface being exposed, and the fundus uteri forming a large tumour on the outside of the vulva

Prolapsus Uteri.

The uterus sometimes leaves its natural situation and falls downwards, so as either to get to the external parts, or out of the body entirely This is most apt to happen when women have a large pelvis, and where the soft parts have been very much relaxed by repeated and severe labours. This disease is called prolapsus uteri, and will be explained more particularly when we come to treat of the diseases of the vagina It is much more frequent than the other disease called the inversio uteri.

Stricture in the Cavity of the Uterus.

A stricture is sometimes formed within the cavity of the uterus, so that its cavity at one part is obliterated entirely. This I believe almost always to take place at one part, viz where the cavity of the fundus uteri terminates, and that of the cervix begins, for in this place the cavity of the uterus is narrowest. As the sides of the cavity round this place lie very near each other, and form naturally a small aperture, it is probable that some slight inflammation may unite the parts together, and shut up the aperture; or the parts may gradually approach' together without this cause, as in strictures of the urethra. The os uteri has been found to be so contracted, as to have its passage in a great measure obliterated ,* and it has even been known to be closed up, by the growth of an adventitious membrane.†

Uterus bony.

The uterus has sometimes its substance more or less converted into bone. This arises from a particular morbid action of its blood vessels, by which they secrete from the

* Vid Morgagni, Epist LXVII. Art. 11.
† Vid. Morgagni, Epist. XLVI. Art. 17.

blood bony matter, and is a very rare disease.

The Uterus changed into an earthy Substance.

The uterus has also been known to be
converted into an earthy substance.* It is
probably of the same kind with the earth
of bones, and this disease probably differs
only from the former, in there being a less
proportion of animal gluten, to combine the
earthy particles together.

A bony Mass in the Cavity of the Uterus.

In the cavity of the uterus a bony mass
is sometimes found. When this is the case,
I suspect that the hard fleshy tubercle
within the cavity of the uterus, such as we
lately described, had been converted into
bone. This at least had taken place in the
only instance which I have known of it,
(for a great part of the tubercle had still

* Vid. Lieutaud, Tom. 1, p. 323.

remained unchanged) and I think it very probable, that it most frequently happens where such bony tumours are found.

Stones in the Cavity of the Uterus.

Stones * have sometimes been found in the cavity of the uterus. These are described by authors as varying in their appearance, some being of a dark, and others of a light colour. About their nature they are silent, and I can say nothing of it from my own knowledge, as it has never occurred to me to see an instance of this disease. I should believe, that these concretions are formed from matter thrown out by the small arteries which open upon the internal surface of the uterus, and are in some degree analogous to the concretions which are formed in some glands of the body.

It has also been known to happen, that a dead foetus has remained for a long time in the cavity of the uterus, and has there

* Vid. Lieutaud, p. 339.

been gradually changed into an earthy mass preserving the shape of the child *

Water in the Cavity of the Uterus

Water has sometimes been known to be accumulated in the cavity of the uterus in very large quantity. * In some cases fifty, sixty, or even a hundred pints, have been said to be accumulated This water is sometimes bloody in its appearance, and at other times is of a yellowish colour. Of its nature I cannot speak particularly, as I have never seen an instance of this disease I should believe, however, from analogy, that the water accumulated in the cavity of the uterus, resembles in its properties the serum , and I should believe also, from the same ground of conjecture, that it is poured out by the small curling arteries of the ute-rus In cases where water is really accu-mulated in the cavity of the uterus, one

* See Cheselden's Anatomy of the Bones, plate LVI.

† Vid Lieutaud, Tom. 1, p. 319 p. 333

must suppose a stricture of the cervix, otherwise the water would escape gradually into the vagina as it is formed. I am apt to believe, however, that where water has been said to be accumulated in the cavity of the uterus, it has frequently been really in large hydatids formed in that cavity.

Hydatids in the Uterus.

Large masses of hydatids* have also been found in the cavity of the uterus. Whether these be of the same kind with what occasionally grow in the placenta, or like those in the other parts of the body, I cannot determine, as it has not occurred to me to see an example of this disease The hydatids of the placenta are a good deal different from those of the liver, kidneys, and some other parts of the body. They consist of vesicles of a round or oval shape, with a narrow stalk to each, by which they adhere on the outside of one another. Some of those hy-

* Vid. Lieutaud, Tom. 1. p 335.

datids are as large as a walnut, and others
as small as a pin's head. A large hydatid
has generally a number of small hydatids
adhering to it by narrow processes Of their
real nature nothing is known, but they are
not improbably animals There is in quadrupeds a difference in hydatids, and this is
even the case in the same species of quadru-
ped; and yet these have been determined to
be animals I should believe that the hydatids said to be found in the uterus, have not
uncommonly been only hydatids of the placenta, which had been retained there.

Rupture of the Uterus.

These are the various diseased appearances which are well ascertained to take
place in the uterus. I have to add, that the
womb is not unfrequently ruptured, which
is rather to be considered as an accident than
a disease. This, perhaps, never takes place
but in the pregnant uterus, and at the time
of delivery. It may arise either from too
violent an action of the muscular fibres of

the uterus upon the child, or upon the hand of an accoucheur, who may for some reason or other have introduced it into its cavity, and pressed upon some part of the uterus with a good deal of force. The ruptures which I have seen have been commonly in the side of the womb, and of considerable extent. The peritonæum covering the womb is often not ruptured, and there is a large mass of black coagulated blood lying between it and the uterus, where the rupture has taken place. This black appearance is occasionally mistaken for mortification.

Two Uteri.

It has sometimes happened, although very rarely, that two uteri have been formed in the same person instead of one In this case there is but one ovarium and one Fallopian tube to each The vagina is at the same time divided by a septum into two canals, each of which conducts to its proper uterus. In the case which is described in the Philosophical Transactions,* a communication was formed at one part through the septum ; but how far this generally takes place in such a kind of monstrosity I cannot determine

The uterus varies a good deal in its size in different persons, in some being fully twice as large as it is in others. It differs also somewhat in the thickness of its substance. There is some difference too in its situation, being often placed much nearer one side of the pelvis than the other. All of these are to be considered as varieties in the natural formation, and not as disease.

* See Philosoph Transact Vol 64, p 474

CHAP. XX.

Diseased Appearances of the Ovaria.

*Inflammation of the Peritonæal Covering of
the Ovaria.*

THAT portion of the peritonæum which
covers the ovaria I believe is seldom inflamed, unless where the inflammation has
spread to it from the uterus, or where it
has attacked this membrane generally. It is
not unusual, however, for it to be inflamed
under either of these circumstances, and it
shews the same appearances as the inflammation of the peritonæum covering any
other part. Adhesions too are frequently
found, joining the ovaria to the neighbouring parts, which had been the consequence
of such an inflammation.

Inflammation of the Substance of the Ovaria.

Where the uterus has been inflamed to a considerable degree, as after parturition, the substance of the ovaria has also been occasionally attacked by the inflammation spreading to it. The ovaria are then enlarged in size, are harder than in a natural state, and are highly vascular ; and very commonly pus is found to have been formed.

Schirrus of the Ovaria.

Schirrus is a disease which sometimes attacks the ovaria, although very seldom in comparison of its attacking the uterus. Under such circumstances the ovaria become enlarged, and are converted into a whitish hard mass, which is more or less intersected with membranous septa These schirrous masses have sometimes a disposition to be converted into bone ; and in this way most frequently, I believe, the ovaria become bony. The bony substance into which they are converted has sometimes a greater admixture of earth than the natural bones of the body.

The ovaria are sometimes very much enlarged in size, and converted into an uniform brown, pulpy matter. Cells are at the same time formed in some part of it which contain a fluid.

I have also seen the ovaria partly changed into a scrofulous matter, intermixed with cells.

Dropsy of the Ovaria.

The most common disease of the ovaria is dropsy. The whole substance of an ovarium is sometimes destroyed, and it is converted into a capsule containing a fluid. These capsules are not unfrequently of a very large size. They consist of a white firm membrane, and contain an aqueous fluid, capable of being partly coagulated.

When the substance of the ovaria is destroyed, and they become dropsical, it is

very common for them to be converted into
a number of cells which communicate with
each other by considerable openings, and to
be prodigiously enlarged in their size. An
ovarium in this case may be so enlarged as
to occupy almost the whole cavity of the
abdomen The ovaria are also sometimes
converted into a congeries of complete cysts.
These vary a good deal in their size, some
being not larger than a hazel nut, and
others as large as an orange. Their coats
are sometimes thin, at other times are of
considerable thickness, and consist of a compact, white, laminated membrane. They
contain either a serous fluid, with which I
have seen some slimy matter mixed, or a
thick ropy fluid, or a kind of jelly ; and,
what one would not expect to find a priori,
different cysts in the same ovarium will
sometimes contain a different sort of fluid.

These cysts, I believe, have been occasionally confounded with hydatids, to which
they bear some resemblance. They are
however really very different They have

much firmer and less pulpy coats than hydatids; they contain a different kind of fluid,
and they are differently connected among
themselves. Hydatids either lie loose with regard to any connection among each other, or
they inclose each other in a series; or small
hydatids adhere to the coats of larger ones.
Cysts of the ovarium adhere to each other
laterally by pretty broad surfaces; do not
envelope each other in a series; and appear
to have no power analogous to generation
like hydatids, by which smaller cysts are
formed, that are attached to those of a
larger size. It appears not improbable,
that these cysts are formed by a gradual
enlargement of the small vesicles which
make a part of the natural structure of the
ovaria.

The Ovaria changed into a fatty Substance with Hair and Teeth.

The ovaria are sometimes converted into
a fatty substance, intermixed with long hair

and teeth, which is surrounded by a capsule consisting of a white strong membrane. The hairs are most of them loose in the fatty substance, but many of them also adhere on the inside of the capsule. Teeth too are formed, but are generally incomplete, the fangs being wanting. These sometimes arise immediately from the inner membrane of the capsule, and are sometimes connected with an irregular mass of bone. Such productions have been commonly considered as very imperfect impregnations, but there is good reason to believe that they can take place without any intercourse between the sexes. I have described a case, which has been published in the Philosophical Transactions, where it was hardly possible that impregnation could have happened. The girl in whom this change of the ovarium was found, could not from all appearances be more than twelve or thirteen years old, the hymen was perfect ; and the uterus had not received that increase of bulk which is usual at puberty. The other marks of puberty were also wanting. From these circumstances I should judge the womb to be incapable of the stimulus of impregnation A tumour, consisting of teeth and hair, was preserved by the celebrated Ruysch * in his collection, which he says was found in a man's stomach. If this be true (which there seems to be no reason to doubt), it puts my conjecture beyond dispute. This production could not possibly, under such circumstances, have any connection with impregnation ; and if it is produced without it in one part of the body, there can be no good reason why it may not also take place without impregnation in another part. These productions are much more frequent in the ovaria than any where else, probably because the process which forms them bears some analogy to generation, in which the ovaria are materially concerned. I must still therefore, whatever objections have been made to it,

* Vid. Ruysch, Tom. 2, Adversar. Anatomicor. Decad. tert.

retain my former opinion. These masses in the ovaria are commonly about the size of a large orange. *

A Fœtus in the Ovarium.

A fœtus is sometimes found in the ovarium This seldom arrives at the full size, but its formation as far as it goes is commonly perfect. When this happens, all vestige of the ovarium is lost, and instead of it there is a bag of some firmness contain-

* I have very lately met with the same kind of fatty substance intermixed with hair, and the body of one tooth covered with enamel, in the ovarium of a young woman about eighteen years of age. In this case the uterus was rather less than its usual size in the adult when unimpregnated, and there was no membrana decidua whatever formed in its cavity It appeared, therefore, to be undergoing no change similar to what happens when there is an ovum growing in the ovarium or the Fallopian tube. The hymen too was perfect, the edge of the membrane being quite sound and natural, and the aperture in it being remarkably small. These circumstances do not amount to demonstrative evidence, but still must be considered as a very strong confirmation of the truth of the opinion above stated.

ing the fœtus, which is attached to the placenta, and is also connected with the chorion that is lying within it. This bag can be ascertained to be the ovarium, by tracing upon it the Fallopian tube and the spermatic vessels, from their origin to their termination. The uterus in such cases is considerably larger than the un-impregnated size, and in its cavity there is formed the membrana decidua. This shews that the uterus takes on the same changes, although imperfectly, which it does in the ordinary circumstances of pregnancy. The spermatic vessels are also enlarged, in order to supply a sufficient quantity of blood to the ovum which is growing in the ovarium.

Shrinking of the Ovaria

The ovaria commonly shrink towards old age, and are changed in their structure. They are diminished to half their natural size, are somewhat tuberculated on their surface, and are very hard. When cut into, the vesicles which make a part of their natural structure, are found to be filled with a white solid matter.

An Ovarium wanting.

An ovarium on one side has been known to be wanting, but this is extremely rare.

CHAP. XXI.

Diseased Appearances of the Fallopian Tubes.

Inflammation of the Fallopian Tubes.

W<small>HEN</small> the uterus is inflamed to a considerable degree, the inflammation not uncom-
monly spreads along the Fallopian tubes :
they become highly vascular, and when
cut open, sometimes contain blood in their
cavities. The inflammation may even advance to suppuration, and their cavities will
be found loaded with pus.

Adhesions.

When the peritonæum generally, or
some part of it, in the neighbourhood of the
Fallopian tubes, is inflamed, the external
covering of these tubes, which is a continu-

ation of the peritonæum, also partakes of the inflammation. This, when it subsides, generally terminates in adhesions of the Fallopian tubes to the contiguous parts. It is not unusual to find the fimbriated extremity of the Fallopian tubes adhering to the ovaria, or when the previous inflammation has been considerable, to find the fimbriated appearance entirely lost, and the body of the Fallopian tube seems to terminate on the surface of the ovarium. Under such circumstances there is no aperture towards this end of the Fallopian tube, and it has lost its power of conveying the ovum from the ovarium to the uterus.

The Fallopian tube communicates by a very small aperture with the cavity of the uterus. This aperture is sometimes obliterated, but not so often as the aperture of that extremity towards the ovarium.

Dropsy of the Fallopian Tubes.

When the Fallopian tube has its aperture closed at both extremities, it is sometimes dilated into a considerable tortuous cavity. This when laid open appears occasionally subdivided by small partial septa, and contains an aqueous fluid, which is capable of being partly coagulated. This fluid is undoubtedly supplied by the secretion of the small arteries belonging to the inner membrane of the Fallopian tube, which is naturally very vascular It may be called dropsy of the Fallopian tube.

The Fallopian Tubes terminating in a Cul-de-sac.

The Fallopian tubes I have seen without any aperture or fimbriated extremity, from a defect in the original formation, and terminating in a cul-de-sac. Under such circumstances they were incapable of per-

T

forming their office as subservient to generation.

An Ovum in the Fallopian Tube.

The Fallopian tube is sometimes dilated into a bag containing an ovum. This arises from the ovum being stopped in its progress from the ovarium to the uterus. When it is so stopped it does not die, but is gradually evolved as if it had been lodged in the cavity of the uterus. This, among many others, is a proof that the uterus is not the only organ which is fitted to evolve an ovum, but that other parts of the body can perform this office. While the ovum is enlarging, the Fallopian tube is more and more dilated, forming a thin bag round the ovum. The blood vessels passing to the ovarium and the Fallopian tube where the ovum is contained, are gradually enlarged, in proportion to the increase of the ovum, in order to supply it with a sufficient quantity of blood While this process is going on in the Fallopian tube, the uterus increases in bulk so as to be even twice its natural size, and becomes more vascular. The cavity of its fundus is also lined by a membrana decidua, and the cervix uteri is plugged up with jelly. The uterus therefore undergoes a variety of changes, exactly similar to what take place in natural pregnancy, being thrown into this progress of action from the original stimulus of impregnation. The ovum sometimes makes considerable progress in the Fallopian tube, and even has been known to advance to the full period of gestation, but more commonly it dies at an early period. In the course of the evolution of the ovum, the Fallopian tube has been known to rupture, and the person to die from internal hæmorrhage. A very clear and accurate account of such a case has been published by Dr. Clarke in the Medical and Chirurgical Transactions *

* See p 216.

T 2

Hard Tumour growing from a Fallopian Tube.

I have seen a hard round tumour growing from the outer surface of one of the Fallopian tubes. This when cut into exhibited precisely the same appearance of structure with the tubercle which grows from the surface of the uterus, viz. it consisted of a hard white substance, which was intersected with strong membranous septa. This, however, I believe to be a very rare appearance of disease.

The round ligaments partake of the inflammation of the uterus, when it is considerable, and has spread to its appendages. They are also, doubtless, subject to other diseases, but these are very rare, and have not fallen under my own observation, nor do I know of their having been particularly noticed by authors.

CHAP. XXII.

Diseased Appearances of the Vagina.

Inflammation of the Vagina.

THE internal surface of the vagina, near the outward opening, is frequently inflamed, especially from the application of the venereal poison, but this hardly ever becomes the subject of examination after death.

Adhesion of the Sides of the Vagina.

A very violent inflammation has sometimes been known to take place in the vagina, which has terminated in the adhesion of the sides of the cavity. This adhesion is sometimes extended over a great part of the cavity, but most frequently is more confined, producing a stricture in some one part. The vagina under such circumstances loses its office as a canal subservient to the uterus; and according to the degree of the extent of the adhesion, the disease becomes more or less easy to be remedied by art.

Ulcers of the Vagina.

Ulcerations are not unusual in the vagina. They sometimes appear like spots of the internal surface, removed as it were by a knife, and at other times there is a foul ragged ulcer. When this last is the case in any considerable degree, the ulcer has commonly not originated in the vagina, but has spread from the womb, which is in a cancerous state. When the ulcer spreads very much, communications are often made with the neighbouring parts, producing a most miserable state of existence. Thus communications are sometimes formed between the vagina and the rectum, or the vagina and the bladder.

Schirrous Tumours in the Vagina.

Schirrous tumours occasionally arise in the vagina itself (although, I believe, rarely) when the uterus is unaffected. When cut into they exhibit the true schirrous structure which has been often described. Such tumours may ulcerate, and produce the same dreadful havock which we have so lately mentioned.

Inversion of the Vagina.

One of the most common diseases of the vagina is its inversion, or prolapsus: this is more apt to happen where the natural formation of the pelvis is large, where the external opening at the vulva is wide, and where the parts are generally relaxed. The prolapsus is more or less in different cases; in some the uterus does not pass out at the external parts, and in others the inversion of the vagina is complete at the extremity

of which is situated the os uteri. The protrusion has then different shapes ; it sometimes forms a large rounded mass, and at
other times it is narrower and more elongated, extending, perhaps, five inches from
the surface of the body.. When this last has
been the case, it has been sometimes mistaken for that species of monstrous formation called hermaphrodite. We may here
take an opportunity of mentioning, that although in some of the common quadrupeds
a real hermaphrodite structure has been
found, yet it has never been discovered
in the human subject When the vagina has
been long in the habit of being inverted, its
inner surface becomes in many parts harder ; it is apt to be inflamed occasionally
from external irritation, and this not uncommonly advances to ulceration.

In inversion of the vagina and prolapsus
of the uterus, if the cavity of the pelvis be
examined, the fundus only of the uterus can
be seen with its appendages very imperfectly, or the whole of the uterus may be

hid entirely: the bladder will then appear to be in contact with the rectum. In this state of the uterus and its appendages, I have known adhesions formed between them and the neighbouring parts. These must have rendered the reduction of the uterus and vagina into their natural situation very difficult, and perhaps till they were a good deal elongated impossible.

The Vagina very short.

The vagina is sometimes very short. I have seen it, I should believe, shorter than half its natural length. This is an original defect in the formation, and can only be very imperfectly remedied by art.

The Vagina widened.

The vagina is sometimes very much stretched or widened by large tumours which are lodged in it: these are chiefly polypi; and when they have been removed by art, the vagina, if it has not been for a long time stretched, recovers nearly its natural size.

The Vagina very narrow.

The vagina has occasionally been found to be very much contracted with regard to transverse diameter, from a defect in the original formation. This, however, occurs very rarely.

CHAP. XXIII.

Diseased or preternatural Appearances of the external Parts.

The Hymen imperforated.

THE hymen is sometimes found without a perforation in it, so that the vagina is completely shut up at its external extremity. This is an original mal-formation, which is frequently not discovered till the age of puberty, when the menstrual blood is accumulated behind it. It is of little consequence, as it can be easily remedied by art.

The Clitoris enlarged.

An enlarged clitoris is also a natural defect, less common than the other, but a more unfortunate one. At birth, the clitoris in such a case is often larger than the penis of a male child of the same age. It has a well formed prepuce and glans, together with a fissure at its extremity, so as to resemble almost exactly the external appearance of the male organs. These cases have given rise to a mistake, with regard to the sex, and females have been often baptized for males. On most occasions, however, where there is an enlarged clitoris, the sex may be determined by the following circumstances. The labia are well formed, and when handled, no round bodies are felt in them, like the testicles. The fissure at the extremity of the glans does not lead to any canal of the urethra, but under the glans, and at the posterior extremity of the fissure, there is an opening which leads immediately to the bladder. I should believe, that by putting a small straight probe into this orifice, and passing it into the bladder, it could be at once determined on most occasions, whether the child was male or female If the child should live to grow up, the clitoris enlarges, but, I believe, not in the same proportion as the penis would do. It is a most unfortunate monstrosity, because it depresses the mind, by a consciousness of imperfect formation in a very important part of the body. Such cases have been often mistaken for hermaphrodites.

The Nymphæ enlàrged.

The nymphæ are not unusually enlarged beyond their natural size. This sometimes happens to one only, and at other times to both. When the nymphæ are very much enlarged, they pass considerably beyond the surface of the body, and have the same sort of covering with the labia, losing by their exposure the fine, vascular, sensible covering of natural nymphæ. This is a monstrous formation of nó great consequence, unless the nymphæ be very large, and even then they can be extirpated by art

The external Labia growing together.

The two external labia are sometimes united together by a fine line of junction, at the upper end of which are situated the meatus urinæ, and the head of the clitoris This sort of monstrous formation is not at all common, and is very easily remedied. When the external labia are separated by a slight operation, all the parts behind are found perfect.

The two labia are sometimes joined together by a continuation of the common skin, so that the appearance of labia is lost entirely. This defect may also be remedied by art, and the parts within will be found to be well formed.

The external parts, particularly the inside of the nymphæ, and the vestibulum, are subject to inflammation and ulcers from common causes, and especially from the application of the venereal poison. These diseases, although they are very often the subject of solicitude during life, yet are seldom examined after death, and therefore we shall omit them here altogether.

CHAP. XXIV.

Diseased Appearances of the Brain and its Membranes.

Inflammation of the Dura Mater

THE dura mater is sometimes found in a state of inflammation. When this is the case, there are to be seen in the inflamed portion of it many extremely fine-vessels, filled with florid blood, which are passing between the dura mater and the cranium. These fine vessels are seldom so crowded as in many other parts of the body when inflamed, which arises from the nature of the membrane itself. In its natural state there are few blood vessels ramifying through it, and therefore when it is inflamed, it does not appear so much crowded with vessels as other parts do which are naturally more

vascular. Still, however, a person well acquainted with the natural appearance of
the dura mater, would be as much struck
with the difference of its appearance when
it is inflamed, as he would be with that of
any other part of the body.

The dura mater during a state of inflammation sometimes forms a layer of coagulable lymph, which adheres upon its inner
surface like an adventitious membrane; but
this is very uncommon On such occasions
although the inflammation of the dura mater may subside, yet the membrane will remain, and may become the cause of a fatal
disease.

When the dura mater is inflamed, adhesions are sometimes formed between it and
the other membranes of the brain, so that
for a considerable extent of surface they
adhere together; but this appearance of disease is also very rare.

It is not uncommon when the dura mater
has been inflamed, especially in consequence
of some external violence, that suppuration

U

takes place, and pus is found covering a portion of the membrane

The dura mater is likewise sometimes eroded by ulceration, but this is by no means frequent : it is more common, in violent injuries of the head, for a portion of it to become mortified.

Scrofulous Tumours connected with the Dura Mater.

Scrofulous tumours are sometimes formed which are connected with the dura mater, but this happens very rarely - These resemble precisely the structure of a scrofulous absorbent gland, and occasionally there is to be found in them a curdly pus.

Spongy Tumours growing from the Dura Mater.

Spongy tumours also grow from the dura mater, but they are very uncommon. Such tumours, as far as I have had an opportunity of examining them, are pulpy to the feeling, and of a distinct fibrous structure.

Bony Matter formed in the Dura Mater.

One of the most common diseased appearances of the dura mater is the formation of bony laminæ in some part of it These are usually very small, being not larger than the nail of a finger, but they are also occasionally of a much larger size. They are thin, and frequently very irregular in their edge. They are not to be found indifferently in every part of the dura mater, but are almost always adhering at the superior longitudinal sinus, or its falciform process In some of them the proportion of the earth to the animal part is larger than in common bone.

There is often but one of these ossifications; at other times there are more of them. The falciform process has been said to be occasionally found almost entirely converted into bone; but this last appearance is very rare

Very strong Adhesion of the Dura Mater to the Cranium.

There is at all times a strong adhesion between the dura mater and the inside of the cranium This adhesion is principally formed by small blood vessels which pass from the one to the other, and likewise by a close application of the fibrous structure of the membrane to the bone In a natural state, however, the dura mater can be perfectly separated from the cranium; yet it sometimes happens that the adhesion is so strong, as to render it impossible to separate the two completely. The dura mater in such an attempt is torn in different parts into two laminæ, one of which adheres to the bone, and the other lies upon the pia mater Whether this preternatural strength

of adhesion arises from a previous state of
inflammation in the dura mater, or from
some other cause, I cannot determine;
but it is not at all an uncommon appearance.

Diseased Appearances of the Tunica Arach-
noides.

Diseased appearances of structure are
very rare in the tunica arachnoides, and have
almost been entirely overlooked by writers.
The only diseased appearance of this coat
which I have observed, is that of its becoming a good deal thicker than it is naturally,
so as to be a pretty firm membrane. In this,
as well as in its natural state, there are to be
seen no blood vessels ramifying upon it, or
at least they are extremely few It is also
separated at some distance from the pia mater, a gelatinous fluid being interposed between the one and the other. This diseased
appearance does not in general take place
equally over the whole surface of the brain,

but is to be found chiefly on the upper part of the two hemispheres. It is not an uncommon appearance of disease, particularly after fevers where the brain has been a good deal affected.

Diseased Appearances of the Pia Mater.

Veins of the Pia Mater turgid with Blood

The most common diseased appearance of the pia mater is that of its veins being turgid with blood. This depends upon some impediment to the free return of the blood from the head towards the heart, which may arise from a variety of causes, and is very different in its appearance from an inflamed state of the pia mater The smaller branches of its arteries, filled with a florid blood, are not more numerous in this state than is natural, but its veins are much more distended with a dark blood.

The Pia Mater inflamed.

When the pia mater is inflamed, it is
upon the whole more difficult to distinguish it from its natural appearance than
any other part of the body. This depends
upon the great number of very small vessels which ramify upon it in its healthy
state. When the pia mater is inflamed, these
small vessels are much more numerous than
in a healthy state, are filled with a florid
blood, and form by their anastomosis a beau-
tiful net-work It does not frequently occur,
when the pia mater is inflamed, that it becomes so uniformly red as to shew no interstices between its vessels, a circumstance
which happens in the inflammation of some
other parts The processes arising from
the under surface of the pia mater are also
more crowded with vessels than usual, and
there is a stronger adhesion between them
and the substance of the brain.

It very rarely happens that any layer

of coagulable lymph is formed in the inflammation of the pia mater, which is so very
common in inflammation of the pleura and
the peritonæum. When the pia mater is inflamed to a high degree, pus is formed. I have
seen pus which had been formed during an
inflammation of the pia mater, and which
was effused over the whole upper surface of ,
the brain

Close adhesions, for some considerable
extent of surface, have been seen between
the pia and dura mater, which are probably the consequence of inflammation ; but
these are very rare, and have not fallen under my own observation.

*Scrofulous Tumours adhering to the Pia
Mater*

I have seen a number of scrofulous tumours adhering upon the inside of the pia
mater   They exhibited the true scrofulous
structure, which has been often explained

This diseased appearance is very uncommon.

It is not unusual to find some of the vessels of the pia mater filled with air. This may be generated by putrefaction, but it is also sometimes seen when no process of this kind appears to have taken place. Under such circumstances, it is probable that air is extricated by some new arrangement in the particles of the blood, somewhat analogous to the change in secretion.

Hydatids.

Little cysts * containing water, (which are generally called hydatids) have been seen adhering to the pia mater; but this is a very rare appearance of disease

* Vid. Lieutand, Tom. 2, p. 145.

Diseased Appearances in the Substance of the Brain.

Inflammation.

The substance of the brain, in which I include both the cerebrum and cerebellum, is liable to inflammation, although it is not very common, when no external injury has been applied to the head. When inflammation takes place, it is rarely extended over any large portion of the brain, but is rather confined to one or more distinct spots In this state of disease the inflamed portion becomes of a red colour, although this is seldom very intense When cut into, the colour is found to arise from a great many small vessels, which are filled with blood If the inflamed portion be upon the surface of the brain, the membranes in the neighbourhood are also commonly inflamed. The part which is inflamed has no peculiar hardness, but yields nearly the same sensation to the touch, as it would do in a healthy state.

Abscesses.

Inflammation of the brain frequently advances to suppuration, and abscesses are formed in it. When these are of a large size, the weight of the pus breaks down the structure of the neighbouring parts, and they look simply as if they had been destroyed, or very much injured by the pressure. When the abscesses are small, there is an ulcerated appearance of the cavity in which the pus is contained

Gangrene.

Portions of the brain occasionally become gangrenous, especially after violent injuries of the head; but I believe this appearance of disease is extremely rare, where an inflammation of the brain has taken place from any other cause I have met, however, with one instance of this; a portion of the brain at the inflamed part was of a very dark brown colour, and as soft as the most rotten pear.

The Brain very soft.

It is extremely common, when a brain is examined in a person who has been dead for several days, to find its substance so soft that it can hardly be cut so as to leave a smooth surface, and the smallest pressure of the fingers breaks it down into a pultaceous mass The brain, however, will sometimes retain, for several days, the firmness and resistance which it had during life; yet this is by no means common Neither of these appearances is to be considered as produced by disease.

The Brain very firm

The brain is sometimes found to be considerably firmer than in a healthy state, to be tougher, and to have some degree of elasticity ;* it will bear to be pulled out with some force, and will re-act so as to re-store itself, or when pressed will recover its former shape. Under such circumstances the ventricles are sometimes found enlarged in size, and full of water. The brain has even been said to become so hard and dry as to be friable between the fingers; and the medullary substance, in these cases, is often much lighter than in a natural state. It has been remarked that the cerebellum is very often unaffected. When these changes take place in the brain, the mind is at the same time deranged : there is either mania, or lethargy, or the person is much subject to convulsive paroxysms.

A white firm Substance formed in the Brain.

It is not a very unusual appearance of

---

* Mr. Hunter is the only person whom I have heard to remark this property of elasticity in the brain of maniacs. It was very remarkable in the only case of this kind which I have had an opportunity of examining.

disease in the brain, to see a part of it changed into a white substance, of an uniform smooth texture, and with a considerable degree of firmness. Around this substance the brain is frequently a little inflamed. Such a substance is generally considered as scrofulous, and it has certainly somewhat that appearance, but it is a good deal firmer than a scrofulous absorbent gland, even where pus has not at all been formed There are frequently more than one of these substances formed in the brain at a time It is also not unusual to find rounded masses of the same sort of substance, lying as it were imbedded in the brain; some of these I have seen as large as a walnut

Encysted Tumours

Encysted tumours containing a serous fluid * have sometimes been found in the substance of the brain ; but they have nevei

* Vid Lieutaud, Tom 2, 194, 195

come under my own observation, and are very uncommon.

Fungous and schirrous Tumours.

Fungous * and schirrous † tumours are also described by authors, as occasionally growing in the brain; but these too are extremely rare. After the operation of the trepan, it is not very uncommon for a fungous tumour to grow from the brain, which is sometimes of a very large size; but what is its particular structure I am unacquainted.

Hydrocephalus.

One of the most common appearances of disease in the brain, is the accumulation of water in its ventricles: this generally takes place when a child is very young, and even sometimes before birth. The

* Vid. Lieutaud, Tom. 2, p 197.
† Vid. Lieutaud, Tom 2, p. 198, 199.

water is accumulated in greater or less
quantity in different cases. It sometimes
amounts only to a few ounces, and occasionally to many pints The water is of a
purer colour, and more limpid, than what
is found in dropsy of the thorax or abdomen. It appears, however, to be of the
same nature with the water that is accumulated in both of those large cavities. In
some trials which I have made, it partly
coagulated upon the application of the
common acids, exactly like the water in
hydrothorax and ascites, or like the serum
of the blood This is not what one-would
expect a priori; it is natural to think, that
as the water which is accumulated in the
ventricles of the brain in a healthy state
does not contain any coagulable matter at
all, or at least in a very small proportion,
there should be the same property belonging to the water when it is accumulated in
a larger quantity, so as to form a disease
This, however, does not necessarily follow,
because the water in hydrocephalus may

not only be supposed to be increased in
quantity beyond what is consistent with
health, but also to be altered in its properties. How far this is always the case in the
water of hydrocephalus, I cannot positively determine. We have no means likewise of ascertaining whether this makes a
part of a general law, with regard to the
accumulation of water in the other circumscribed cavities of the body, or whether it
is an exception to it. In the cavities of the
abdomen, thorax, &c. there is just enough of
moisture, in the healthy state, to lubricate
the surfaces of parts, and it cannot become
an object of chemical examination, till it is
accumulated beyond the healthy proportion, so as to form a disease. We can make
no comparative trials, therefore, between
the one fluid and the other.

When water is accumulated in the ventricles to a very large quantity, the substance of the brain, especially upon the sides
and at the upper surface, appears almost to
be a sort of pulpy bag, containing a fluid.

X

The scull too upon such occasions is very much enlarged in size, and altered in its shape The cranium is exceedingly large in proportion to the size of the face The projections are very considerable at the centres of ossification, from whence the frontal, parietal, and occipital bones were originally formed, and the membranous divisions between these several bones are very wide. When the scalp is removed, so as to give an opportunity of looking immediately upon the cranium, the bones are found to be very thin, often not thicker than a shilling, and there are frequently broad spots of membrane in the bone The reason of this last appearance is, that ossification takes place in many points of the membrane in such cases in order to make a quicker progress, but the water accumulates too rapidly for it, so that spots of membrane are left not converted into bone When such appearances take place in hydrocephalus, the disease has been of long continuance, occasionally for some years.

Water is also sometimes formed under the pia mater, and upon the surface of the brain, but very rarely in any considerable quantity. There is, generally, at the same time a greater quantity than natural in the ventricles.

Water is likewise found in small quantity between the dura and pia mater.

It is related by authors, that water has been formed occasionally between the dura mater and the cranium.* From the nature of the adhesion between the cranium and this membrane one would not easily be led to suspect an accumulation of water between them, and such cases are at least to be considered as very uncommon.

Blood effused or extravasated.

Blood is frequently found effused within the cavity of the cranium in various situations. It may either be poured out by the rupture of some vessel into the substance of

* Vide Lieutaud, Tom. 2, p. 229, 230.

X 2

the brain itself, or into some of the ventricles. It is frequently effused upon the surface of the brain under the pia mater, and likewise between the dura and the pia mater. This is most apt to happen where the effusion is in consequence of external violence. The quantity of blood which is effused from the rupture of vessels in the brain is frequently very considerable. It is commonly found in a coagulated state, and the texture of the brain in the neighbourhood is often very much hurt from the pressure. When blood is extravasated within the cavity of the cranium from some external injury, the vascular system is usually sound, except for the rupture which may have happened. But when blood is extravasated within the cavity of the cranium where there has been no external injury, the vascular system of the brain will be almost always found diseased. It is very common in examining the brain of persons who are considerably advanced in life, to find the trunks of the internal carotid arteries upon the side of the sella turcica very much diseased, and this disease extends frequently more or less into the small branches. The disease consists in a bony or earthy matter being deposited in the coats of the arteries, by which they lose a part of their contractile and distensile powers, as well as of their tenacity. The same sort of diseased structure is likewise found in the basillary artery and its branches.

The vessels of the brain under such circumstances of disease, are much more liable to be ruptured than in a healthy state. Whenever blood is accumulated in unusual quantity, or the circulation is going on in them with unusual vigour, they are liable to this accident, and accordingly in either of these states, ruptures frequently happen. Were the internal carotid arteries and the basillary artery not subject to the diseased alteration of structure which we have described, effusions of blood within the cavity of the cranium, where there has been

no previous external injury, would be very
rare.

Diseased Appearances of the Plexus Choroides.

The plexus choroides seems to be subject
to some diseases to which the vascular system of the brain generally is very little or
not at all exposed.

Its vessels become sometimes a good deal
enlarged and varicose.

Little bags resembling hydatids sometimes adhere to it. These are commonly
small, viz. not larger than a garden pea,
but sometimes they have been seen as large
as a gooseberry.

Small scrofulous tumours sometimes adhere to the plexus choroides ; but this is a
much rarer appearance of disease than the
former.

Earthy Matter in the Pineal Gland.

There is but one sort of disease to which the pineal gland is much exposed, and this is very frequent: it consists in a deposition of earthy matter in its substance. It very rarely happens that a pineal gland is entirely free from earth, but it is occasionally almost entirely converted into it. There is then a very thin covering of the natural substance of the pineal gland surrounding an earthy mass, and the mass itself is always very easily divisible into small particles, by pressure between the fingers.

The pineal gland has been mentioned by some authors as being sometimes schirrous. I have felt it on some occasions a little firmer than on others; but it has never occurred to me to observe that alteration of structure in it which could be properly called schirrous, and I believe it to be a very rare disease. The pineal gland has been found to be very much distended with

a limpid water ;* but this too is very uncommon.

That particular substance called the
glandula pituitaria is liable to very few
diseases ; I have never seen in it any decided or obvious alteration from its natural
structure. It is somewhat firmer in one
person than another, but this never struck
me to be disease.

It rarely happens that any of the nerves
within the cavity of the cranium appear
diseased. I have, however, sometimes seen
a nerve a good deal smaller in its size than
it ought to be, softer in its texture, and of
a less opaque colour ; this I recollect to
have been particularly the case with one of
the optic nerves in a person who was blind
of one eye.

The nerves vary a good deal in their size
in different persons, as a part of their original formation, without there being any
disease whatever.

These are the principal diseased changes

* Vid. Morgagni, Epist LXII. Art. 15.

which take place in the brain, and its appendages. I have just to add, that the
brain is subject to great variety from original monstrous formation. A great part of
what is usually called the cerebrum is sometimes wanting, while the cerebellum, and the
medulla spinalis are entire ; sometimes there
is hardly any vestige of either the cerebrum
or cerebellum, and the medulla spinalis is
very much diminished in size ; at other
times there is a total want of the brain, and
there is no appearance of the medulla spinalis. In this case one should expect a
want of nerves through the whole body. It
is, however, not so ; nerves are found distributed in the common way, through the
limbs, and the dorsal nerves can be seen
arising from a membrane somewhat resembling the dura mater in the canal behind
the vertebræ. When there is a total want
of brain, it sometimes happens that there is
a medulla spinalis, which, however, is of
a very diminished size. In cases of deficiency in the brain, the cranium is nearly

upon a level with the two eyes, and there is often upon the scalp a soft spongy excrescence. This is generally divided into distinct protuberant masses, and is covered with a fine skin, capable of being rendered very vascular by injection When cut into, the spongy excrescence consists of pretty large cells, which are filled with a sort of grumous matter.

There is also frequently, instead of this excrescence, a bag growing from the skin of the scalp, and covering more or less the back of the trunk. This bag sometimes consists of a fine membrane, with little strength, at other times it is pretty thick, and has very considerable firmness It sometimes communicates with the cavity of the cranium by a considerable opening; and at other times the communication is very small. It is filled with an aqueous fluid, and in some instances there is also in it a portion of the brain

FINIS.

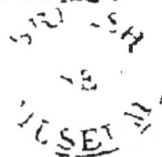

Lightning Source UK Ltd.
Milton Keynes UK
UKHW052054120121
376916UK00009B/1577

9 781140 843351